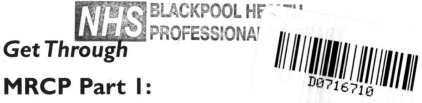

Get Through

MRCP Part 1:
1000 Best of Fives

The Blackpool F

I would like to dedicate this book to Professor John M. Porter MD

Get Through

MRCP Part 1: 1000 Best of Fives

Second Edition

Una Coales MD FRCSEd FRCSOto DRCOG DFFP MRCGP
GP, London, UK

Editorial Adviser

Eric Beck FRCP
*Emeritus Physician, Whittington Hospital; PDS Academic Lead,
Royal Free and University College Medical School, London, UK*

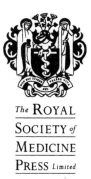

The ROYAL
SOCIETY *of*
MEDICINE
PRESS Limited

© 2004 Royal Society of Medicine Press Ltd

Published by the Royal Society of Medicine Press Ltd
1 Wimpole Street, London W1G 0AE, UK
Tel: +44 (0)20 7290 2921
Fax: +44 (0)20 7290 2929
E-mail: publishing@rsm.ac.uk
Website: www.rsmpress.co.uk

British Library Cataloguing in Publication Data
A catalogue record for this book is available from the British Library

ISBN 1-85315-579-9

Distribution in Europe and Rest of World:
Marston Book Services Ltd
PO Box 269
Abingdon
Oxon OX14 4YN, UK
Tel: +44 (0)1235 465500
Fax: +44 (0)1235 465555

Distribution in the USA and Canada:
Royal Society of Medicine Press Ltd
c/o Jamco Distribution Inc
1401 Lakeway Drive
Lewisville, TX 75057, USA
Tel: +1 800 538 1287
Fax: +1 972 353 1303
E-mail: jamco@majors.com

Elsevier Australia
30–52 Smidmore Street
Marrickville, NSW 2204
Australia
Tel: + 61 2 9517 8999
Fax: + 61 2 9517 2249
E-mail: service@elsevier.com.au

Phototypeset by Phoenix Photosetting, Chatham, Kent
Printed in the UK by Bell & Bain, Glasgow

Contents

Preface

The completion of the transformation of the MRCP (UK) Part 1 examination into two papers of 100 questions each, using the single best answer multiple choice format (BOF or Best of Five), necessitates a new edition of this book.

This gives the opportunity not only to convert previous true/false MCQs into BOFs, a task requiring skill and ingenuity, but also to create completely new up-to-date questions. As a result 400 new BOFs have been added to the 600 of the previous edition; the latter have been reviewed and, in some cases, revised.

The 1000 BOFs have been arranged in ten test papers. Each question is graded on a three-point scale of difficulty from which is calculated a notional pass mark for the whole paper. This means that the pass mark will vary from a difficult paper (e.g. 59%) to an easy paper (e.g. 72%). It also means that every candidate meeting this standard will pass, so variations in pass rate can occur. This reflects the principle of criterion referencing now used in the MRCP (UK) examinations.

A glossary of abbreviations used, where not always explained in the text, has been added.

The book has been written in collaboration with Dr Eric Beck, a former examiner of the Royal Colleges of Physicians, who has had many years' experience of examining in the clinicals and (now defunct) orals, setting written questions and participating in the construction of the current MRCP examination.

Eric Beck
Una Coales
ufcmd@aol.com

Recommended texts and references

American Psychiatric Association (2000) *Diagnostic and Statistical Manual of Mental Disorders*, 4th edn. American Psychiatric Association, Washington D.C.

Beck E. *et al.* (2003) *Tutorials in Differential Diagnosis*, 4th edn. Churchill Livingstone, London.

Braunwald E. *et al.* (2001) *Harrison's Principles of Internal Medicine*, 15th edn. McGraw-Hill, New York.

Brooks G.R. *et al.* (2001) *Jawetz Melnick Adelberg's Medical Microbiology*, 22nd edn. Appleton & Lange, Connecticut.

*Champe P.C. *et al.* (1994) *Lippincott's Illustrated Reviews: Biochemistry*, 22nd edn. Lippincott-Raven.

Collier J.A.B. *et al.* (2003) *Oxford Handbook of Clinical Specialties*, 6th edn. Oxford University Press, Oxford.

Fitzpatrick T.B. *et al.* (2001) *Color Atlas and Synopsis of Clinical Dermatology*, 4th edn. McGraw-Hill, New York.

*Ganong W.F. (2003) *Review of Medical Physiology*, 21st edn. Medical Books/McGraw-Hill.

GMC Publications such as *Good Medical Practice* and *Duties of a Doctor* are essential reading and obtainable free by downloading from the website: www.gmc_uk.org

Greenhalgh T. (2001) *How to Read a Paper*, 2nd edn. BMJ Books, London.

Hoffbrand A.V. *et al.* (2001) *Essential Haematology*, 4th edn. Blackwell Scientific Publications, Oxford.

Longmore M. *et al.* (2001) *Oxford Handbook of Clinical Medicine*, 5th edn. Oxford University Press, Oxford.

Jenkins R. *et al.* (2004) *WHO Guide to Mental Health in Primary Care*, The Royal Society of Medicine Press, London.

Kumar P.J. *et al.* (2002) *Clinical Medicine*, 5th edn. Baillière Tindall, London.

McMinn R.M.H. (1994) *Last's Anatomy Regional and Applied*, 9th edn. Churchill Livingstone, London.

MRCP (UK) Part 1 Examining Board (2002) *Part 1 Syllabus*, Royal College of Physicians, London.

MRCP (UK) Part 1 Examining Board (2003) *MRCPUK Part 1 Papers 2002*, Royal College of Physicians, London.

Royal Pharmaceutical Society of Great Britain (2003) *British National Formulary 46*. British Medical Association, London.

Rubenstein D. *et al.* (2003) *Lecture Notes on Clinical Medicine*, 6th edn. Blackwell Scientific Publications, Oxford.

The Editorial Board (2001) *Advanced Life Support Course Provider Manual*, Resuscitation Council (UK), London.

Tomb, D.A. (1999) *Psychiatry*, 6th edn. Lippincott, Williams and Wilkins, Baltimore.

Website of MRCP(UK) Central Office provides up to date information: http//www.mrcpuk.org

*Contains single best answer MCQs

List of abbreviations

ACE	angiotensin-converting enzyme
ACTH	adrenocorticotrophic hormone
ADH	antidiuretic hormone
A&E	Accident and Emergency
AFB	acid fast bacilli
AIDS	acquired immune deficiency syndrome
ALP	alkaline phosphatase
ALT	alanine aminotransferase
ANA	antinuclear antibody
ANCA	antineutrophil cytoplasm antibody
APS	autoimmune polyglandular syndrome
APTT	activated partial thromboplastin time
ARDS	adult respiratory distress syndrome
ARR	absolute risk reduction
AST	aspartate transaminase
AV	atrioventricular
AZT	azidothymidine
BMI	body mass index
BNF	British National Formulary
BSE	bovine spongioform encephalopathy
C	complement
CA	cancer antigen
CD	cluster designation
CJD	Creutzfeldt–Jakob disease
CK	creatine kinase
COPD	chronic obstructive pulmonary disease
CRP	C-reactive protein
CSF	cerebrospinal fluid
CT	computed tomography
CVP	central venous pressure
DDAVP	1-deamino-8-D-vasopressin
DEXA	dual-energy X ray absorptiometry
DKA	diabetic ketoacidosis
DLCO	carbon monoxide diffusion in the lung
DS-DNA	double-stranded deoxyribonucleic acid
ECG	electrocardiogram, -graphy
EEG	electroencephalogram, -graphy
EM	electron microscopy
ERCP	endoscopic retrograde cholangiopancreatography
ESR	erythrocyte sedimentation rate
FEV_1	forced expiratory volume in 1 second
FiO_2	fractional concentration of oxygen in inspired gas
FOB	faecal occult blood
FSGS	focal segmental glomerulosclerosis
FSH	follicle-stimulating hormone
FTA	fluorescent treponemal antibody
FVC	forced vital capacity
G6PD	glucose-6-phosphate dehydrogenase

GBM	glomerular basement membrane
GCS	Glasgow coma scale
GGT	γ-glutamyltransferase
GI	gastrointestinal
GTN	glyceryl trinitrate
HAART	highly active antiretroviral treatment
Hb	haemoglobin
HBcAg	hepatitis B core antigen
HBeAg	hepatitis B e antigen
HBsAg	hepatitis B surface antigen
HCG	human chorionic gonadotrophin
HCV	hepatitis C virus
HDL	high density lipoprotein
5-HIAA	5-hydroxyindoleacetic acid
HIV	human immunodeficiency virus
HLA	human leucocyte antigen
HOCM	hypertrophic obstructive cardiomyopathy
HRT	hormone replacement therapy
HSMN	hereditary motor and sensory neuropathy
HSP	Henoch–Schönlein purpura
IDDM	insulin dependent diabetes mellitus
IF	immunofluorescence
Ig	immunoglobulin
IHD	ischaemic heart disease
INR	international normalised ratio (of prothrombin time)
ITP	idiopathic thrombocytopenic purpura
JVP	jugular venous pressure
K	potassium
KCO	diffusion coefficient
KUB	(plain x-ray film of) kidneys, uretus and bladder
LBBB	left bundle branch block
LDH	lactate dehydrogenase
LDL	low density lipoprotein
LH	luteinising hormone
LVH	left ventricular hypertrophy
MAOI	mono amine oxidase inhibitor
MCV	mean corpuscular volume
MEN	multiple endocrine neoplasia
MI	myocardial infarction
MRCP	magnetic resonance cholangiopancreatography
MRI	magnetic resonance imaging
Na	sodium
NIDDM	non insulin dependent diabetes mellitus
NNT	number needed to treat
NSAIDs	non steroid anti-inflammatory drugs
OR	odds ratio
OSA	obstructive sleep apnoea
PAN	polyarteritis nodosa
PAWP	pulmonary artery wedge pressure
PCO_2	partial pressure of carbon dioxide
PCR	polymerase chain reaction

PCV	packed cell volume
PEG	percutaneous endoscopic gastrostomy
PO_2	partial pressure of oxygen
PRV	polycythaemia rubra vera
PT	prothrombin time
PTC	percutaneous transhepatic cholangiogram, -graphy
PTH	parathyroid hormone
PUVA	phototherapy with ultra violet A
RBBB	right bundle branch block
RCT	randomised control trial
RNA	ribonucleic acid
RTA	renal tubular acidosis or road traffic accident
SIADH	syndrome of inappropriate ADH secretion
SLE	systemic lupus erythematosus
SVC	superior vena cava
T_3	tri-iodothyronine
T_4	thyroxine
TB	tuberculosis
TCA	tricyclic antidepressant
TLC	total lung capacity
TPA	tissue plasminogen activator
TSH	thyroid-stimulating hormone
TT	thrombin time
VDRL	venereal disease reference laboratory
VIP	vasointestinal peptide
VMA	vanillylmandelic acid
VT/VF	ventricular tachycardia/ventricular fibrillation
WCC	white cell count
WPW	Wolff–Parkinson–White

INTRODUCTION

THE MRCP (UK) EXAMINATION 2004 sees the completion of the implementation of the recommendations made in the major review of the examination in 1997.
The changes relating to the **PART ONE** examination are:

Part 1 syllabus:
First published by the MRCP (UK) Central Office in November 1999 and to be regularly updated.
MCQ PAPERS ONE and TWO (3 hours each)
  100 STEMS each with 5 answers from which ONLY ONE is selected giving 100 TRUE (100 marks)

Composition of papers
The two papers will together contain 200 questions broken down under the following headings. They will be randomised across the two papers:

Cardiology		15
Clinical Haematology & Oncology		15
Clinical Pharmacology, Therapeutics & Toxicology		20
Dermatology		8
Endocrinology		15
Gastroenterology		15
Infections & Sexually Transmitted Diseases		15
Nephrology		15
Neurology		15
Opththalmology		4
Psychiatry		8
Respiratory Medicine		15
Rheumatology		15
Clinical Science:		25
Cell, molecular and membrane biology	2	
Clinical anatomy	3	
Clinical biochemistry and metabolism	4	
Clinical physiology	4	
Genetics	3	
Immunology	4	
Statistics, epidemiology & evidence based medicine	5	
		===
		200

Negative marking
An incorrectly selected answer will not be given a negative mark (−1). (Thus guessing is no longer penalised!)

Criterion referencing
The difficulty of each question will be assessed by a panel of experts and a notional score agreed. The sum of the ease and

difficulty of questions will determine the **PASS MARK** for that paper and all candidates achieving it will pass. So the easier the paper the higher the pass mark and vice versa.

THIS BOOK incorporates all the changes in the **PART ONE** examination and will help you prepare for it by providing:

10 complete **PART ONE** papers each comprising 100 BEST OF FIVE (BOF) MCQs. The composition of each paper will follow the **CONTENT** and **SEQUENTIAL ORDER** of questions as in the actual examination but not quite so rigidly.

The 1000 BOFs will cover a substantial part of the syllabus. The same topics, but in a different format, may occur in more than one paper occasionally, as in the actual examination; for example, a particular stem might generate three separate sets of questions on investigation, diagnosis and treatment. If these were to appear as three consecutive questions in one paper, they could be so inter-related as to cue the candidates to the correct answer for all three or, conversely, an incorrect answer to the first might falsely cue the other two.

The **ANSWER KEY** to the questions is annotated to explain some of the more difficult answers. Each question will be **CRITERION REFERENCED** using a three point scale of how difficult or easy a candidate just passing the whole examination would find that particular question:

* 25–50% "just passing" candidates expected to get correct
** 50–75% "just passing" candidates expected to get correct
*** 75–100% "just passing" candidates expected to get correct.

Remember that "guessing" gives you a 20% (one-in-five) chance of being correct.

The overall profile of the make up of each paper can then be translated into a NOTIONAL pass mark for each paper (**this is purely a guide for the candidate and may differ from the method of calculation in the actual examination**).

The pass mark in the new ten 100 BOF MCQ papers ranges between 59 and 72 out of a possible 100 marks (see Table 1). Remember you are required to select **ONE** completion only in each BOF and there is **ONE** mark for the correct answer; as is implied in the appellation BOF the four distractor completions should be plausible partly correct answers but will attract no marks.

Table 1: Criterion Referencing

	*	**	***	Notional Pass Mark %
Paper 1	14	48	38	69
Paper 2	11	39	50	72
Paper 3	14	37	49	71
Paper 4	7	60	33	69
Paper 5	14	49	37	68
Paper 6	8	57	35	69
Paper 7	24	43	33	65
Paper 8	35	45	20	59
Paper 9	30	41	29	62
Paper 10	10	48	42	71

(see text for definition of starring system)

Advice on answering BOFs

However childish it may sound the first advice given to examination candidates in their school days still holds good:

READ THE QUESTION CAREFULLY BEFORE ANSWERING IT.

Question setters try very hard to avoid ambiguity in the terms they use and candidates should be aware of the meaning of frequently used wordings:

CHARACTERISTIC:	if not present would make you unsure of the diagnosis
RECOGNISED:	does happen but may be uncommon
MOST/MAJORITY:	over 50%
CAN/MAY:	a correct answer
ALWAYS/NEVER:	usually an incorrect answer as medicine, like life, rarely has certainties; setters usually therefore avoid these words
LONG ANSWERS:	often tend to be correct – but not always.

Look out, particularly in BOFs, for questions requiring ONE NEGATIVE answer e.g. "all the following are correct except".

The ordering of completions A to E is increasingly in alphabetical order unless it upsets the sense of the question.

Make sure you are familiar with the system of transcribing your answers into the boxes on the mark sheet. Use the 2B pencil provided and rub out thoroughly any you consider on review, to have entered incorrectly.

With the abolition of negative marking there is now a positive incentive against leaving answers blank so try and answer each BOF.

When selecting the best one in a BOF rather than weighing each answer against the other four see if you can decide what you would have given as the best answer unprompted and check whether this appears amongst the five offered – you are more likely to be right. This format can however mean that the best answer sometimes will not be listed if it is obviously so superior to all the others (which would turn the question into a best of one!) This is not as easy when you are asked to choose a "negative" in a format such as: "all the following answers are correct EXCEPT ...". The question, in effect, becomes a WORST OF FIVE! Do not be confused by such negative formatting – again, READ THE QUESTION CAREFULLY BEFORE ANSWERING IT.

3

MRCP Paper One BOFs

In these questions candidates must select one answer only

Questions

1. A 50-year-old diabetic woman presents with fever and a dusky red erythematous eruption over the left side of her face. The MOST likely organism would be

   A Staphylococcus aureus
   B Group B streptococcus
   C Group A streptococcus
   D Herpes zoster virus
   E Herpes simplex virus

2. A 23-year-old woman complains of an offensive green vaginal discharge. On examination she has an inflamed cervix. The MOST useful investigation is

   A Gram stain of an endocervical swab
   B wet film of a high vaginal swab
   C darkfield microscopy
   D virology on an endocervical swab
   E pH of a high vaginal swab

3. The MOST appropriate antibiotic would be

   A amoxicillin 3 g stat
   B doxycycline 100 mg bd for 7 days
   C ciprofloxacin 500 mg as a single dose
   D metronidazole 400 mg bd for 5 days
   E clotrimazole pessary 500 mg as a single application

4. A 22-year-old HIV-positive Ugandan man being treated with a protease inhibitor presents with hypopigmented anaesthetic annular lesions with raised erythematous rims and painful nodules on his legs. On examination, a thickened ulnar nerve is palpated at the elbow and running into the lesions. He is also noted to have multiple transverse white lines on his fingernails. The MOST appropriate treatment would be

A standard TB treatment, discontinue the protease inhibitor and use alternative anti-retroviral drugs until the TB has been treated
B dapsone
C prednisolone
D rifampicin and dapsone
E benzylpenicillin

5. A 17-year-old boy presents with pain on swallowing. On examination he has trismus, palatal petechiae and enlarged tonsils. His sclerae are jaundiced. The MOST likely causative organism is

A *Streptococcus pneumoniae*
B hepatitis B virus
C Epstein–Barr virus
D herpes simplex virus
E *Clostridium tetani*

6. A 36-year-old pregnant woman presents with high fever, jaundice, vomiting and drenching sweats. She had returned from Brazil a month ago. On examination she is also noted to have hepatosplenomegaly. Her test results are as follows

White cell count	11.5×10^9/L
Hb	↓8.0 g/dL
Platelets	100×10^9/L
Plasma glucose	↓3 mmol/L
Plasma sodium	↓130 mmol/L
Plasma potassium	↓3.6 mmol/L
Plasma creatinine	↑180 µmol/L

The MOST useful diagnostic investigation is

A Dengue fever serology
B microscopy of thick blood film with Giemsa stain
C Mantoux test
D blood cultures
E Lassa fever serology

7. The SINGLE factor giving rise to a poorer prognosis would be

A white cell count
B plasma creatinine level
C age
D pregnancy
E anaemia

8. Lymphatic filariasis (*Wuchereria bancrofti*) is associated with all of the following EXCEPT

A blindness
B elephantiasis
C conjunctival loa loa
D urticaria
E pulmonary infiltrates

9. A 23-year-old female with Hodgkin's disease presents with small, white mucosal flecks in her mouth that can be wiped off. The MOST likely diagnosis is

A lichen planus
B candidiasis
C aphthous ulcers
D squamous cell carcinoma
E infectious mononucleosis

10. A 20-year-old healthy man presents with acute shortness of breath, fullness in the head and blackouts. He smokes 10 cigarettes a day and drinks socially. He is noted to have a ruddy plethora, JVP 6 cm and dilatation of veins on his chest wall. Diagnosis is BEST confirmed by

A bronchoscopy and biopsy
B chest x-ray
C lymph node biopsy
D thoracic CT scan
E bone marrow aspirate

11. A 40-year-old woman presents with fatigue, dyspnoea and paresthesiae. On examination she has a red tongue. Her blood film shows hypersegmented neutrophils, a Hb 9 g/dL and an MCV 120 fl. The MOST likely diagnosis is

A vitamin B_{12} deficiency
B iron deficiency
C coeliac disease
D sideroblastic anaemia
E hypothyroidism

12. A 20-year-old woman presents with recurrent epistaxis. She admits to having heavy periods. Blood pressure is 90/60 and her pulse 100. There are bruises of different ages over her extremities but no splenomegaly. Her test results are as follows

White cell count 8×10^9/L
Hb   ↓11.5 g/dL
Platelets   ↓20×10^9/L
Bleeding time   ↑prolonged
Antinuclear antibody negative ANA (−ve)

The MOST likely diagnosis is

A non-accidental injury
B systemic lupus erythematosis
C idiopathic thrombocytopenia
D thrombotic thrombocytopenic purpura
E sickle cell disease

13. A 40-year-old man presents with fever, sweating and weight loss. On examination he is noted to have splenomegaly. Blood test results

White cell count   ↑100×10^9/L with neutrophilia
Hb   ↓11 g/dL
Platelets 200×10^9/L
Plasma uric acid   ↑500 μmol/L (210–480)
Plasma alkaline phosphatase   ↑500 IU/L (30–300 IU/L)
Serum B12   ↑1 nmol/L (0.13–0.68 nmol/L)
Leucocyte alkaline phosphatase low

The MOST likely diagnosis is

A chronic lymphocytic leukaemia
B chronic myeloid leukaemia
C acute myeloid leukaemia
D acute lymphoblastic leukaemia
E septicaemia causing leukaemoid reaction

14. The following statements regarding testicular tumours are correct EXCEPT

A Seminomas usually present in men in their 40s.
B Teratomas are radiosensitive.
C Cryptorchism is a risk factor.
D The contralateral testicle should be biopsied if there is a history of infertility.
E After orchidectomy the disease is staged by chest and abdominal CT scan.

15. A 30-year-old man presents with a tender swollen testicle. He states that he was hit in the groin while playing football. On examination, the borders of the testicle are irregular, and the testicle is heavy and woody. There is no associated lymphadenopathy. He is also noted to have gynaecomastia. There are no external signs of trauma. In this age group, the MOST likely diagnosis is

A testicular torsion
B epididymo-orchitis
C seminoma
D teratoma
E testicular haematoma

16. A 70-year-old man presents with bone pain and severe gout. On examination he is noted to have a large tongue, and a tender left calf with a large non-infective necrotic ulcer. Blood test results

plasma calcium	↑ 3.9 mmol/L
alkaline phosphatase	↑ 300 IU/L (30–300 IU/L)
plasma urea	↑ 10 mmol/L
plasma creatinine	↑ 300 µmol/L
ESR	↑ 50 mm/h

The BEST test to confirm the diagnosis is

A serum uric acid
B bone marrow examination
C biopsy ulcer
D urine electrophoresis
E bone scan

17. A 20-year-old man back from hitchhiking through South America 2 weeks previously now presents with explosive, watery, foul-smelling diarrhoea and weight loss. On examination, he has abdominal distension. His stools are greasy and contain mucus. The MOST appropriate treatment would be

A ciprofloxacin
B prednisolone
C metronidazole
D oral rehydration
E pancreatic enzyme supplements

18. A 40-year-old woman on carbamazepine for trigeminal neuralgia now complains of severe dizziness. The other medication she might be taking that may have potentiated the effects of carbamazepine is

   A combined oral contraceptive pill
   B erythromycin
   C chloramphenicol
   D omeprazole
   E thiazide diuretics

19. A 35-year-old indigent man is taking long-term anti-tuberculous chemotherapy. He now complains of itching and diarrhoea. He has poor memory and emotional blunting, making it difficult to understand him. The MOST likely diagnosis is

   A chronic renal failure
   B pellagra
   C liver disease
   D drug allergy
   E scabies

20. An 87-year-old man is noted to have an altered level of consciousness. The serum glucose is 37 mmol/L with a serum sodium of 163 mmol/L. He has no prior history of diabetes. He has been on intravenous fluids for a week with IV cefuroxime and metronidazole for a chest infection. The MOST appropriate treatment would be

   A insulin sliding scale, heparin and 0.45% saline
   B insulin sliding scale, heparin and 0.9% saline
   C insulin sliding scale, 0.9% saline
   D insulin sliding scale, 0.45% saline
   E insulin sliding scale, dextrose saline

21. A 40-year-old actor with insulin-dependent diabetes mellitus is started on propranolol for stage fright. He collapses on stage. He has not changed his insulin regime. His glucose is 1.5 mmol/L. The MOST beneficial advice you would offer him after treatment would be

   A discontinue propranolol
   B carry a chocolate bar
   C decrease his Humulin insulin
   D decrease his Actrapid insulin
   E carry glucagon

22. A 50-year-old schizophrenic presents with drooling saliva and involuntary chewing movements. He walks with a shuffling gait. The MOST likely diagnosis is

A Parkinson's disease
B extrapyramidal side-effect of medication
C autonomic side-effect of medication
D anticholinergic side-effect of medication
E lithium toxicity

23. A 50-year-old farmer presents with acute shortness of breath, dizziness and severe headache. His skin is red in colour, and he smells of bitter almonds. He mentions that he had been using rodenticides. His condition rapidly deteriorates. The MOST likely agent that is poisoning him is

A cyanide
B arsenic
C organophosphate
D warfarin
E paraquat

24. A 45-year-old male psychiatric patient with long-term bipolar disorder presents with vomiting, muscle twitching and tremor. He was started on bendrofluazide recently and self-prescribes ibuprofen for headaches. Blood pressure 90/50. His gait is ataxic. He then has a series of epileptic fits. The drug MOST likely to be responsible is

A lithium
B phenothiazine
C benzodiazepine
D ecstasy (methylenedioxy methamfetamine)
E ibuprofen

25. You are on ward rounds and notice that a young patient is coughing briskly. He has just been commenced on benzylpenicillin for acute tonsillitis complicated by trismus. He states he does not know if he is allergic to any drugs. He becomes short of breath. His pulse is 110 beats/minute and he now cannot complete sentences. The MOST appropriate management for this patient would be

A administer 0.5 ml adrenaline (epinephrine) of a 1:10,000 solution intravenously for suspected anaphylaxis

B administer 0.3 mg adrenaline intramuscularly for suspected new-onset asthma attack

C administer oxygen at 15 L/min and give nebulised salbutamol 5 mg for suspected severe asthma attack

D administer oxygen at 15 L/min and 0.5 ml adrenaline of a 1:1000 solution intramuscularly for suspected anaphylaxis

E administer oxygen at 10 L/min and give IV hydrocortisone 200 mg immediately for anaphylactic shock

26. A 20-year-old man presents with ingestion of paraquat-containing pesticide 2 hours prior. The MOST appropriate initial management is

A 100% oxygen and urine test to confirm paraquat absorption

B tracheal intubation

C gastric lavage followed by activated charcoal therapy and tracheal intubation

D oral administration of repeated-dose activated charcoal with magnesium sulphate every 4 hours until charcoal is seen in the stool

E haemodialysis

27. A 22-year-old man presents with fever 1 hour after his first injection of benzylpenicillin therapy for primary syphilis. He complains of headache, muscle pains and chills. On examination: pulse 110, respiratory rate 20/min and blood pressure 100/60. White cell count is $12.5 \times 10^9/L$ with neutrophilia. The MOST likely explanation is

A Jarisch–Herxheimer reaction

B drug anaphylaxis

C neurosyphilis

D meningitis

E HIV-conversion illness

28. A 50-year-old man complains of difficulty in hearing and dyspnoea. He is noted to have a nasal septal perforation and a blood pressure of 140/90. His urinalysis shows red cells, protein and casts. The chest-x-ray reveals opacities. The MOST likely diagnosis is

A tuberculosis
B amyloidosis
C Goodpasture's syndrome
D acute tubulointerstitial nephritis
E Wegener's granulomatosis

29. A 13-year-old girl presents with a painful and swollen knee. There is no history of trauma. A tender lump is palpated over the tibial tuberosity. The MOST likely diagnosis would be

A osteomyelitis
B chondromalacia patella
C juvenile rheumatoid arthritis
D osteosarcoma
E apophysitis of the tibial tubercle (Osgood–Schlatter disease)

30. A 40-year-old woman complains of disabling joint pains. On examination you note scaly plaques over her anterior shins and knees. She has tried diclofenac for the arthralgia and wonders if there is any connection with the rash. The MOST useful treatment for her joints now would be

A oral prednisolone
B methotrexate
C co-dydramol
D topical 0.5% hydrocortisone
E dithranol 0.1% cream

31. A 40-year-old woman complains of intolerance to cold weather and cold running water. On examination you note she has a beaked nose, radial furrowing of the lips and facial telangiectasiae. On examination of her hands you notice sausage-like digits and tapered fingers. The MOST discriminating investigation to establish her diagnosis is

A anticentromere antinuclear antibody
B rheumatoid factor
C full blood count
D chest x-ray
E barium swallow

32. A 15-year-old girl presents with fever and red, hot, swollen wrists and knees. On examination there is a diastolic mitral murmur not heard again later during her admission and a pink ring-shaped rash with slightly raised edges on the trunk. Initial blood results show a raised ESR and leukocytosis. The MOST likely diagnosis is

A gonorrhoea infection
B systemic lupus erythematosus (SLE)
C rheumatic fever
D infective endocarditis
E juvenile rheumatoid arthritis (Still's disease)

33. A 20-year-old man presents with buttock pain radiating down both legs and heel pain. On examination he has marked kyphosis and limitation of chest expansion. ESR and CRP are raised. The MOST likely diagnosis is

A lumbar disc prolapse
B sacro-illitis
C spondylolisthesis
D spinal stenosis
E ankylosing spondylitis

34. A 44-year-old woman complains of headaches and nosebleeds. Blood pressure is 160/100 in the right arm and 130/80 in the left arm. She complains of cold legs. The MOST likely diagnosis would be

A acromegaly
B Marfan's syndrome
C coarctation of the aorta
D Kawasaki's disease
E Takayasu's arteritis

35. A 50-year-old man presents to A&E complaining of 30 minutes of severe crushing mid-chest pain with no relief from GTN. He has a history of angina. His pulse is 105 and his BP 115/60. The 12-lead ECG shows normal sinus rhythm only. The FIRST drug to administer would be

A morphine
B oxygen
C gaviscon
D streptokinase
E atropine

36. A 40-year-old woman with a history of angina presents with severe chest pain for 30 minutes. Her pulse is 45 and her blood pressure 80/60. Her ECG shows second-degree heart block. The FIRST drug to administer would be

A lidocaine (lignocaine)
. B atropine
C adrenaline (epinephrine)
D procainamide
E amiodarone

37. A 40-year-old patient is brought to Casualty by ambulance in pulseless electrical activity (PEA). You are told he was given adrenaline (epinephrine). The NEXT step would be to

A evaluate for reversible causes
B cardiovert with 200J shock
C administer verapamil
D administer amiodarone
E administer morphine

38. A 30-year-old drug addict is noted to have a pansystolic murmur heard best at the bottom of his sternum. Giant "cv" waves are present in the jugular venous pulse. The MOST likely diagnosis would be

A ventricular septal defect
B atrial septal defect
C mitral regurgitation
D tricuspid regurgitation
E pulmonary stenosis

39. A woman in the 29th week of pregnancy collapses in a crowded casualty waiting room. She is not breathing and has no palpable pulse when seen by the SHO. The MOST appropriate initial management is

A Call for help, place the patient in the supine position and commence CPR until the crash trolley arrives.

B Call for help, for the crash trolley and the obstetrician on call, place the patient on a trolley with a pillow under the right buttock and flank and commence CPR.

C Call for the cardiac arrest team, obstetric and paediatric registrar on call, place the patient on a trolley with a pillow under the left buttock and flank and commence CPR until the crash trolley arrives.

D Call for help, place the patient on a trolley with a pillow under the right buttock and flank, and wheel the patient straight up to labour ward for an emergency Caesarean section.

E Call for help – cardiac arrest team and for the obstetric and paediatric registrars on call, place the patient on a trolley with a pillow under the right buttock and flank, wheel the patient into the resuscitation room, give 100% oxygen, continue CPR until the defibrillator ECG leads are attached and a rhythm confirmed.

40. A 55-year-old man has been treated with three consecutive shocks of 200, 200 and 360 Joules for ventricular fibrillation. The morphology of his rhythm does not change. The MOST appropriate next step in management is

A administer 4th shock at 360 Joules immediately

B recheck pulse and administer 4th shock at 360 Joules

C recheck pulse and administer amiodarone 300 mg IV if the systolic BP is <90

D recheck pulse and blood pressure, commence CPR and administer lignocaine 50 mg if the systolic BP is <90

E recheck pulse and blood pressure, commence CPR and administer amiodarone 300 mg IV if the systolic BP is >90

41. A 55-year-old farmer complains of dry cough, exertional dyspnoea, joint pains and weight loss. He is noted to have finger clubbing. On x-ray there are bilateral diffuse reticulonodular shadowing at the bases. The MOST likely diagnosis is

A bronchial carcinoma

B bronchiectasis

C cryptogenic fibrosing alveolitis

D mesothelioma

E extrinsic allergic alveolitis

42. An 18-year-old known asthmatic presents with severe wheezing and a respiratory rate of 30 and a pulse of 120. She is using her accessory muscles and appears distressed. She is apyrexial. The MOST appropriate initial management would be

A IM adrenaline (epinephrine)
B oxygen and nebulised salbutamol
·C IV dexamethasone
D endotracheal intubation
E IV penicillin

43. A 25-year-old woman is brought to Casualty by ambulance having sustained gross maxillofacial deformities following a high speed RTA. She is now agitated and hypoxic despite high-concentration oxygen having been administered by face mask by the paramedics. The MOST appropriate immediate intervention is

A endotracheal intubation
B nasopharyngeal airway
C oropharyngeal airway
D cricothyroidotomy
E laryngeal mask airway

44. A 14-year-old boy with cystic fibrosis presents with pneumonia. He also suffers from mild renal failure. The MOST appropriate antibiotic treatment is

A tobramycin and carbenecillin
·B ciprofloxacin
C tetracycline
D erythromycin
E cephalosporin

45. A 70-year-old alcoholic man presents with sudden onset of productive purulent cough. The chest x-ray shows consolidation of the left upper lobe. The MOST likely pathogen is

A *Staphylococcus aureus*
B *Streptococcus pneumoniae*
C *Klebsiella pneumoniae*
D *Mycoplasma pneumoniae*
E *Pseudomonas aeruginosa*

46. A 40-year-old longstay patient in a psychiatric hospital presents with fever, abdominal pain, dry cough and worsening confusion. Blood tests reveal neutrophilia, lymphopenia and hyponatraemia. Chest x-ray shows right-sided lobar consolidation. The MOST likely diagnosis is

A tuberculosis
B *Streptococcus pneumoniae*
C *Legionella pneumoniae*
D *Klebsiella pneumoniae*
E *Staphylococcus pneumoniae*

47. A 60-year-old priest presents with cough, dyspnoea, dull chest pain and vague epigastric pain. On examination the left chest shows diminished expansion, stony dull percussion note and absent breath sounds. There is aegophony at the apex. The mediastinum is shifted to the right. The chest x-ray confirms a unilateral pleural effusion. A pleural tap shows

Specific gravity	1.020
Total protein	↑40 g/L
LDH	↑300 IU (70–250 IU/L)
Amylase	↑300 Somogyi U/dL (0–180 Somogyi U/dL)

Possible diagnoses include the following EXCEPT

A acute pancreatitis
B pancreatic pseudocyst
C lung cancer
D oesophageal rupture
E tuberculosis

48. The MOST appropriate management for this patient is

A lie the patient flat and refer urgently to ophthalmologist
B sit the patient upright and refer urgently to ophthalmologist
C place the patient at a 45 degree angle and refer urgently to ophthalmologist
D prescribe IV acetazolamide (diamox) and refer urgently to ophthalmologist
E arrange for urgent Doppler scan of the carotid

49. A football player presents with a drop foot after receiving a kick to his right leg. He can neither dorsiflex nor evert the foot. Sensation is lost over the front and outer half of the leg and dorsum of the foot. The MOST likely diagnosis is injury to

A superficial peroneal nerve
B common peroneal nerve
C tibial nerve
D lateral popliteal nerve
E sural nerve

50. A 50-year-old diabetic man presents with a unilateral facial nerve palsy and severe earache. On auroscopic examination, he has granulation tissue deep in the external auditory meatus. The MOST likely diagnosis is

A Bell's palsy
B sarcoidosis
C facial nerve schwannoma
· D otitis externa complicated by local osteomyelitis (malignant otitis externa)
E suppurative otitis media

51. A 40-year-old man presents with progressive confusion and tremor. On examination, he has extensor plantar reflexes. The MOST useful investigation would be

A HIV serology
B computerised tomography (CT scan)
C drug screen
D Mantoux test
, E VDRL

52. A 45-year-old man with a history of epilepsy presents with several weeks of fluctuating levels of consciousness. On examination his pupils are unequal. The MOST discriminating investigation is

A HIV serology
• B computerised tomography (CT scan)
C electroencephalogram (EEG)
D drug levels
E lumbar puncture

53. A 23-year-old woman complains of general fatigue, muscle ache and double vision. On examination you note ptosis, but the pupils are equal, round and reactive. She tires easily from talking. The MOST discriminating investigation would be

A thyroid function tests
B antinuclear antibody
C smooth muscle antibody
D lumbar puncture
E anti-acetylcholine receptor antibodies

54. A 60-year-old hypertensive presents with a painful right eye. On examination he is noted to have right partial ptosis and right fixed dilated pupil. The eye is looking downwards and outwards. The MOST likely diagnosis is

    A trochlear nerve palsy
    B abducens nerve palsy
    C incomplete oculomotor nerve palsy
    D posterior communicating artery aneurysm
    E optic neuritis

55. A 50-year-old man complains of stabbing pains in his chest and calves. He walks with a wide-based gait. On examination he has ptosis and small, irregular pupils. He has absent knee jerk reflexes. The MOST likely diagnosis is

    A subacute combined degeneration of the cord
    B syringomyelia
    C tabes dorsalis
    D Friedreich's ataxia
    E multiple sclerosis

56. A 40-year-old man presents with numbness and tingling sensation in his feet. He is noted to have distal sensory loss and absent ankle jerk reflexes. The knee-jerk reflexes are exaggerated. He drinks heavily and smokes cigars. Blood pressure 160/90 with a pulse of 90. Full blood count reveals a macrocytic anaemia. The MOST likely diagnosis is

    A syringomyelia
    B tabes dorsalis
    C Wernicke–Korsakoff syndrome
    D vitamin B_6 deficiency
    E subacute combined degeneration of the cord

57. A 60-year-old man presents acutely with vertigo and vomiting. On neurological examination there is right facial numbness, an ipsilateral ataxia of arm and leg and a contralateral loss of pain and temperature sense. The MOST likely diagnosis is an ischaemic lesion in the territory of

    A posterior cerebral artery
    B middle cerebral artery
    C anterior cerebral artery
    D posterior inferior cerebellar artery
    E vertebrobasilar ischaemia artery

58. A 60-year-old man presents with headache and gradual loss of central vision and loss of red/green discrimination. He is being treated with atenolol for hypertension and has just been diagnosed as having pernicious anaemia. He drinks 4 units of alcohol a week and smokes 20 cigarettes a day. The MOST likely diagnosis is

A basilar migraine
B cerebral tumour
• C tobacco amblyopia
D central retinal artery occlusion
E central retinal vein occlusion

59. An 80-year-old woman complains of sudden painless loss of vision in her right eye. She has facial pain on chewing. The MOST likely diagnosis is

A acute glaucoma
B retinal detachment
• C cranial arteritis
D basilar migraine
E optic neuritis

60. A 25-year-old man presents to Casualty with an alkaline chemical injury to his eyes. He complains of burning eyes. On examination he has white eyes with blanched out blood vessels (limbal ischaemia). The MOST appropriate treatment would be

A apply local anaesthetic and irrigation with sterile H_2O
B test pH with litmus paper and neutralise with acid
• C refer urgently to ophthamology specialist
D apply local anaesthetic and sweep the conjunctiva with a cotton bud
E place the head of the patient in a filled sink of water

61. A 40-year-old diabetic complains of seeing flashing lights and floaters in his eye. On examination he is noted to have a unilateral irregular field defect. The MOST likely diagnosis is

A migraine with focal aura
B vitreous haemorrhage
• C retinal detachment
D acute angle closure glaucoma
E central retinal artery occlusion

62. A 40-year-old woman complains of double vision, worse at night. She had a similar episode 10 years ago that resolved spontaneously. Her visual acuity is worse in the right eye and colours appear less bright. Her vital signs are normal. The MOST discriminating investigation is

 A fundoscopic examination
 B MRI scan
 C slit lamp examination
 D lumbar puncture
 E antinuclear antibodies

63. A 20-year-old heroin addict presents with weight loss, diarrhoea and confusion. On examination he has purple papules on his legs. The MOST useful investigation is

 A echocardiogram
 B blood cultures
 C HIV serology
 D chest x-ray
 E drug levels

64. A 20-year-old slightly withdrawn man states he experiences auditory hallucinations. He is noted to have poverty of speech and a flat affect. The MOST likely diagnosis would be

 A schizophrenia
 B manic-depressive disorder
 C delirium
 D dementia
 E opioid abuse

65. A 70-year-old man presents with confusion. On examination he is noted to have fixed pupils, nystagmus and an inability to look outwards. He has a broad-based gait. The MOST likely diagnosis is

 A Marchiafava–Bignami syndrome (degeneration of the corpus callosum)
 B Wernicke–Korsakoff syndrome
 C lateral medullary syndrome
 D tabes dorsalis
 E vitamin B_{12} deficiency

66. A 60-year-old alcoholic man presents with confusion and unsteadiness for several weeks. Blood pressure is 190/110 and pulse 60. His pupils are unequal and his reflexes generally brisk. The MOST likely diagnosis is

A epidural haematoma
·B subdural haematoma
C subarachnoid haemorrhage
D Wernicke–Korsakoff syndrome
E viral encephalitis

67. A 50-year-old man with a history of previous myocardial infarction presents to Casualty with chest pain. Initial blood pressure is 110/70. During evaluation, he collapses. ECG shows ventricular tachycardia. He has no palpable pulse. The MOST appropriate management would be

A synchronised DC shock at 100J
B administer IV amiodarone 150 mg over 10 mins
°C DC cardioversion with 200J
D administer IV lidocaine (lignocaine) 50 mg over 2 mins
E commence CPR

68. A 70-year-old woman presents with progressive dysphagia and food regurgitation. On examination she has halitosis and a small lump on the left-side of her neck.

The MOST likely diagnosis is

A achalasia
B branchial cyst
C diffuse oesophageal spasm
D pharyngeal pouch
E myasthenia gravis

69. A 50-year-old man presents in shock with rigors and a temperature of 40°C. He is jaundiced and is tender on palpation of the liver, which is felt 5 cm below the costal margin. Dark concentrated urine is noted upon Foley catheter insertion. The FIRST investigation would be

A liver function tests
°B blood cultures
C abdominal ultrasound
D hepatitis A, B and C virology
E endoscopic retrograde cholangiopancreatography (ERCP)

70. A 55-year-old woman complains of sudden severe central abdominal pain radiating to her back and vomiting. She prefers to sit forwards on her stretcher. Temperature is 39°C, BP 100/60 and pulse 112. On examination she has a markedly tender epigastrium and a bruise over the left flank. She has a history of gallstones. She denies smoking or alcohol. She takes HRT. The MOST discriminating investigation would be

A plain abdominal x-ray
B serum bilirubin and liver function tests
C serum amylase
D full blood count
E abdominal ultrasound

71. A 60-year-old man presents with increasing abdominal girth. On examination you elicit shifting dullness. You decide to obtain an ascitic fluid tap. The following should be routinely requested on the fluid EXCEPT

A cell count
B Gram stain and culture for bacteria and AFB
C albumin and protein
D cytology
E glucose

72. A 45-year-old woman presents with severe itching, recent pale stools and dark urine. On examination there is darkened skin pigmentation, xanthelasma and hepatomegaly. Her test results are:

Serum bilirubin   15 µmol/L
Serum alkaline phosphatase ↑400 IU/L (30–300 IU/L)
AST   ↑40 IU/L (5–35 IU/L)

The SINGLE best test to confirm the diagnosis is

A serum antimitochondrial antibody
B hepatitis virology
C liver biopsy
D Kveim test
E abdominal ultrasound

Paper One BOFs questions

73. A 60-year-old man presents with increasing abdominal girth. On examination you elicit shifting dullness. The ascitic fluid tap reveals straw-coloured fluid containing 50 g/L of protein and elevated LDH. It contains 1000 WBC/mm³ (no lymphocytes) and many red cells are present. His serum total protein is 40 g/L. The MOST likely diagnosis is

  A cirrhosis
  B tuberculosis
  C malignancy
  D pancreatitis
  E hepatic vein obstruction

74. A 55-year-old man complains of rectal bleeding. He is noted to have freckles on his lips. His father had undergone bowel surgery but he is not sure why. The MOST likely diagnosis is

  A Crohn's disease
  B ulcerative colitis
  C Peutz–Jegher syndrome
  D hereditary haemorrhagic telangiectasia
  E familial adenomatous polyposis

75. A 40-year-old woman presents with a right-sided pleural effusion and ascites. Abdominal ultrasound reveals a left ovarian mass. The MOST likely diagnosis is

  A pseudomyxoma peritonei
  B Meig's syndrome
  C Budd–Chiari syndrome
  D nephrotic syndrome
  E tuberculosis

76. A 44-year-old woman presents with fatigue and ascites. She is noted to have an irregular pulse of 120 with small volume. The chest x-ray is unremarkable. The 12-lead ECG demonstrates atrial fibrillation with low QRS voltage and T-wave inversion. The MOST likely diagnosis is

  A right heart failure due to mitral stenosis
  B Budd–Chiari syndrome
  C constrictive pericarditis
  D primary pulmonary hypertension
  E tuberculous peritonitis

77. A 50-year-old woman presents with watery diarrhoea and right iliac fossa pain. On examination a rumbling mid-diastolic murmur is auscultated at the lower left sternal border, louder on inspiration, and the liver is enlarged. 12-lead ECG shows peak, tall P waves in lead II. The MOST useful investigation would be

A serum gastrin
B urine 5-hydroxy-indole acetic acid (5HIAA)
C serum vasoactive intestinal peptide (VIP)
D urine vanillyl-mandelic acid
E fasting calcium

78. A 60-year-old man presents with persistent fever, profuse watery diarrhoea and crampy abdominal pain for the past week. He has just completed treatment for osteomyelitis. Proctosigmoidoscopy reveals erythematous ulcerations and yellowish-white plaques. The MOST likely diagnosis is

A ulcerative colitis
B Crohn's disease
C pseudomembranous colitis
D viral gastroenteritis
E Clostridium perfringens enterocolitis

79. A 40-year-old woman presents with abdominal bloating, diarrhoea and weight loss for 9 months. She had last felt really well on holiday in Tunisia over a year ago. Results show:

White cell count	11×10^9/L
Hb	9 g/dL
Platelets	150×10^9/L
Blood film	microcytes and macrocytes, hypersegmented neutrophils Howell-Jolly bodies

The MOST likely diagnosis is

A Crohn's disease
B tropical sprue
C coeliac disease
D giardiasis
E Whipple's disease

80. A 66-year-old woman presents in a coma. Temperature 35°C, pulse 50 and BP 140/80. On examination she has a goitre and few basal rales in the chest. Her deep tendon reflexes are not brisk. Her medications are thyroxine, bendrofluazide and omeprazole. Blood results:

Plasma sodium   ↓129 mmol/L
Plasma potassium ↓ 3.6 mmol/L
Plasma urea   10 mmol/L
Plasma creatinine   130 μmol/L
Plasma glucose   ↓ 3 mmol/L

The MOST appropriate medication would be

A naloxone
B furosemide (frusemide)
• C triiodothyronine
D dextrose infusion
E hydrocortisone sodium succinate

81. A 16-year-old girl presents with an anterior neck mass. It moves on protrusion of her tongue. Thyroid radionucleotide scan shows no uptake in the midline. The MOST likely diagnosis is

A lingual thyroid
B Hashimoto's thyroiditis
• C thyroglossal cyst
D thyroid follicular adenoma
E Riedel's thyroiditis

82. A 50-year-old woman who underwent a thyroidectomy a week ago now presents with confusion. She also complains of perioral tingling. The MOST discriminating investigation is

A serum glucose
B liver function tests
C full blood count and film
D thyroid function tests
• E serum calcium

83. A 60-year-old man presents to Casualty drowsy and confused. Blood test results:

Serum sodium   ↑150 mmol/L
Serum potassium   ↑5 mmol/L
Serum chloride   105 mmol/L
Serum bicarbonate   30 mmol/L
Serum urea   10 mmol/L
Serum glucose   ↑40 mmol/L

The following management is advisable EXCEPT

A 0.9% saline IVI
B heparin
C insulin at 3 U/h
D measure serum potassium hourly
E blood cultures

84. A 50-year-old man complains of loss of libido. He takes Humulin and Actrapid insulin. He is noted to have an enlarged liver. The MOST discriminating investigation is

A serum copper and caeruloplasmin
B serum gamma-glutamyl transferase
C HbsAg
D serum iron and total iron binding capacity
E mitochondrial antibodies

85. An 18-year-old female, who recently started the combined oral contraceptive pill on holiday in Kenya, complains of colicky abdominal pain, vomiting and fever. She develops progressive weakness in her extremities. The MOST likely diagnosis is

A acute pyelonephritis
B acute intermittent porphyria
C ureteric calculus
D malaria
E systemic lupus erythematosis

86. A 20-year-old female presents with acne and hirsutism. She complains of a year of chaotic menstrual cycles with long periods of amenorrhoea. She has gained weight recently. She has never been pregnant. On examination there are no other abnormalities. The MOST appropriate initial investigation would be

A laparoscopy
B 24-hour urinary free cortisol
C serum 17-hydroxyprogesterone levels
D serum LH, FSH and testosterone levels
E chromosome karyotyping

87. A 45-year-old obese man is noted to have glycosuria. He has no symptoms. Diabetes is confirmed on oral glucose tolerance test. The MOST appropriate management for this patient is

A commence biguanide
B commence sulphonylurea
•C advise on diet and exercise
D commence on Humulin and Actrapid insulin
E admit to hospital

88. A 60-year-old woman presents with a firm nodular midline neck mass. Blood tests reveal the presence of antibody to thyroglobulin and low serum thyroxine. The CORRECT diagnosis is

A Grave's disease
B deQuervain's thyroiditis
C Riedel's thyroiditis
•D Hashimoto's thyroiditis
E thyroid carcinoma

89. A 70-year-old woman presents with recent onset of urinary incontinence. The MOST appropriate initial investigation is

•A MSU for dipstick
B urodynamic studies
C full blood count
D serum urea and electrolytes
E MSU for culture and sensitivities

90. A 65-year-old diabetic man presents with a painless distended bladder. His urine dipstick shows no evidence of infection. The MOST useful investigation is

A excretion urography
B retrograde ureterography
C serum urea and electrolytes
D cystourethroscopy
•E pressure-flow studies

91. A 40-year-old man presents with proteinuria, haematuria and progressive renal failure. He is also noted to have a high frequency sensorineural hearing loss. He has a sister who was noted to have microscopic haematuria but is asymptomatic. The MOST likely diagnosis is

A membranous glomerulonephritis (GN)
•B Alport's syndrome
C Goodpasture's syndrome
D Wegener's granulomatosis
E focal glomerulosclerosis

92. A 60-year-old man presents with fits and confusion. He has a past history of myocardial infarction and bowel resection. On chest examination there are bilateral rales and crackles. There has been no urine output from his Foley catheter. His serum urea is 50 mmol/L and his potassium is 8 mmol/L. The FIRST MOST appropriate step would be

A 15 units of soluble insulin with 50 g glucose (50%) IV
◦B 10–30 ml IV calcium gluconate (10%)
C continuous arteriovenous haemofiltration
D haemodialysis
E bicarbonate (100 mls of a 4.2% solution) by IVI

93. A 45-year-old well-controlled insulin-dependent diabetic had been prescribed captopril for hypertension. He has a history of intermittent claudication and suffers rest pain. There is now 3+ proteinuria and urea and creatinine are elevated. On examination there is an abdominal bruit. The MOST likely diagnosis for his renal condition is

A diabetic nephropathy
B focal segmental glomerulosclerosis
◦C renal artery stenosis
D membranous glomerulonephritis
E renal cholesterol embolism

94. A 50-year-old woman presents with flaccid bullae over her trunk and limbs. She takes penicillamine and diclofenac for her rheumatoid arthritis. The MOST likely diagnosis for her skin condition is

A bullous pemphigoid
◦B pemphigus vulgaris
C epidermolysis bullosa
D dermatitis herpetiformis
E systemic lupus erythematosus

95. A 60-year-old woman presents with a slowly-growing, painless but itchy flat red scaly plaque on her lateral lower calf. The MOST useful investigation would be

A skin scrapings
◦B skin biopsy
C serum glucose
D none – spot diagnosis
E sentinel node biopsy

96. Stevens–Johnson syndrome is associated with all of the following drugs EXCEPT

A penicillin
B sulphonamides
• C oral contraceptives
D thiazide diuretics
E salicylates

97. A 65-year-old farmer presents with a grey thickened patch of skin on the rim of his left ear. The 1-cm lesion is painless, raised, firm, and has not changed in size over many years. The MOST likely diagnosis is

A basal cell carcinoma
B keratoacanthoma
• C solar keratosis
D seborrhoeic keratosis
E squamous cell carcinoma

98. A 20-year-old man presents with a brown discoloured toenail. On examination there is nail pitting and brown pigmentation at the base of the great toe-nail and the cuticle. He states that the colour started under the nail and has spread down to his nail-bed. The MOST likely diagnosis is

A subungual haematoma
B psoriasis
C paronychia
• D melanoma
E onychomycosis

99. A 30-year-old woman presents with a solitary painless genital ulcer with a hard, indurated base. The MOST useful investigation of the lesion is

A Gram stain
• B dark field microscopy
C virology
D saline mount
E biopsy

100. A 20-year-old man complains of urethral discharge and lesions on his palms and penis. He also complains of itchy burning eyes and pain in his right knee. On examination you note crusty scaling papules on his palms and glans penis. Subungual cornified material is seen but no nail pitting. The MOST likely diagnosis is

A gonorrhoea infection
B Reiter's syndrome
C Behçet's syndrome
D chlamydia infection
E psoriasis

Answers to Paper One BOFs

Criterion Referencing Marks

*   – 25–50% of candidates expected to get correct
**   – 50–75% of candidates expected to get correct
***   – 75–100% of candidates expected to get correct

The notional PASS MARK is 69%

---

1. C *** The rash is erysipelas.

2. B *** *Trichomonas vaginalis* is associated with a "strawberry" cervix. Wet film demonstrates the flagellated organism.

3. D *** The treatment for *Trichomonas vaginalis* infection is metronidazole.

4. B * Rifampicin should be avoided in the presence of anti-retroviral drugs.

5. C *** This boy has infectious mononucleosis (glandular fever).

6. B ** The patient has malaria.

7. D **

8. D **

9. B ***

10. C ** The diagnosis of Hodgkin's disease is best made by lymph node biopsy. Bronchoscopy in the presence of SVC obstruction to evaluate for bronchial carcinoma is ill-advised.

11. A ***

12. C ***

13. B **

14. B ** Seminomas are radiosensitive.

15. D **

16. B ** The patient has multiple myeloma.

17. C *** This man most likely contracted giardiasis from contaminated water. Diagnosis is made on stool microscopy for cysts or trophozoites. Serology may also be positive.

18. B *

19. B ** Isoniazid is associated with B_6 deficiency.

20. A ***

21. A ** Propranolol has a hypoglycaemic effect and also masks the autonomic response to hypoglycaemia.

22. B ***

23. A *** Warfarin is used in rat poison.

24. A **

25. D *

26. D *

27. A **

28. E ***

29. E *

30. B * She has psoriatic arthropathy.

31. A *** This woman most likely has progressive systemic sclerosis (CREST).

32. C ** On examination the disappearing murmur is known as the Carey-Coombs murmur.

33. E ***

34. C **

35. B ***

36. B **

37. A **

38. D ***

39. E **

40. E **

41. C ***

42. C ***

43. D *

44. B **

45. C **

46. C ** This organism is common in institutions, in hotels, etc. with ventilation systems.

47. E ** All the options produce pleural exudates but tuberculosis is the only one not associated with increase in amylase.

48. A *

49. B ** The common peroneal nerve may be injured at the neck of the fibula.

50. D *

51. E ** The patient has syphilis.

52. B ** The patient has a subdural haematoma.

53. E *** This woman most likely has myasthenia gravis.

54. D **

55. C ***

56. E *** The patient has vitamin B_{12} deficiency.

57. D *** Also known as lateral medullary syndrome.

58. C * This is a case of optic atrophy induced by tobacco due to cyanide poisoning and exacerbated by vitamin B_{12} deficiency.

59. C *** Also known as temporal arteritis, blood should be taken for an ESR and prednisolone commenced immediately.

60. C * This patient has limbal ischaemia and warrants urgent ophthamologist referral as the patient is at risk of corneal necrosis in <24 hours!

61. C **

62. B ** MRI is likely to show patchy demyelination characteristic of multiple sclerosis.

63. C *** The patient has Kaposi's sarcoma.

64. A ***

65. B **

66. B ***

67. C *** Pulseless ventricular tachycardia is a shockable rhythm.

68. D ***

69. B **

70. C *** Grey–Turner's sign is associated with acute pancreatitis.

71. E **

72. A *** This woman most likely has primary biliary cirrhosis.

73. C **

74. C **

75. B ***

76. C ***

77. B *** This woman presents with carcinoid syndrome. 24h urinary excretion at >15 mg of 5-HIAA is diagnostic. CT scan and laparotomy may also be indicated.

78. C ***

79. C **

80. C ** This patient has myxoedema coma.

81. C **

82. E *** This patient most likely has hypocalcaemia as a complication of thyroid surgery and injury to the neighbouring parathyroid glands.

83. A ** 0.45% saline should be used if the Na is >150.

84. D ** This man may have haemochromatosis.

85. B *

86. D ** This woman most likely has polycystic ovarian disease.

87. C **

88. D ***

89. A ***

90. E **

91. B **

92. B **

93. C ** ACE inhibitors should be avoided in silent atherosclerosis, in particular, renal artery stenosis and may precipitate acute renal failure if administered.

94. B ** Pemphigus vulgaris is precipitated by penicillamine.

95. B ** The lesion is probably Bowen's disease.

96. C **

97. C **

98. D *

99. B * The patient has a syphilitic chancre.

100. B ***

MRCP Paper Two BOFs

In these questions candidates must select one answer only

Questions

1. A 23-year-old female with Hodgkin's disease presents with small, white mucosal flecks in her mouth that can be wiped off. The MOST appropriate management for this patient would be

   A betamethasone valerate cream
   B acyclovir
   C penicillin
   D oral nystatin
   E biopsy before initiating any of the above

2. A 30-year-old man with HIV presents with sudden bilateral painless loss of vision. The MOST likely cause is

   A Kaposi's sarcoma
   B histoplasmosis
   C *Chlamydia trachomatis*
   D CMV retinitis
   E gonococcal infection

3. The organism MOST frequently isolated from the ascitic fluid of patients with spontaneous bacterial peritonitis is

   A *Streptococcus milleri*
   B *Escherichia coli*
   C *Streptococcus pneumoniae*
   D *Bacteroides fragilis*
   E *Pseudomonas aeruginosa*

4. A 20-year-old HIV-positive man presents with fever and meningism. CSF shows:

Pressure	250 mmH$_2$O
WBCs	200/mm^3
Predom. Cells	lymphocytes
Glucose	33% plasma level
Protein	5 g/L

You suspect cryptococcal meningitis. Diagnosis is BEST confirmed by

A India ink stain of CSF
B CSF cryptococcal antigen
C culture of CSF
D blood culture
E Gomori methenamine-silver staining of culture

5. A 20-year-old college student presents with headache, ear ache and dry cough. The chest x-ray shows left lower lobe consolidation. White cell count is normal. The MOST likely pathogen is

A *Streptococcus pneumoniae*
B *Klebsiella* sp.
C *Mycoplasma pneumoniae*
D *Haemophilus influenzae*
E *Legionella pneumophila*

6. A 17-year-old girl presents with meningism and conjunctival petechiae. The CSF is turbid with an abundance of polymorphs and protein. Gram-negative cocci are isolated. The MOST likely organism is

A *Neisseria meningitidis*
B *Neisseria gonorrhoea*
C Group B streptococcus
D *Haemophilus influenzae*
E *Streptococcus pneumoniae*

7. A 22-year-old woman, back from Thailand a fortnight ago, is rushed to casualty in a comatose state. On examination she is jaundiced and unrousable. Her reflexes are exaggerated. Blood results show:

White cell count	4.0×10^9/L
Hb	4 g/dL
Blood film	asexual forms, parasite count 10% of rbc's
PCV	12%
Creatinine	265 μmol/L
Bilirubin	40 μmol/L
Blood glucose	2 mmol/L
Arterial blood gas	pH 7.2, HCO_3 12 mmol/L
Lactate	6 mmol/L

The MOST likely diagnosis is

A yellow fever
B trypanosomiasis
C *Plasmodium falciparum* malaria
D *Plasmodium ovale* malaria
E *Plasmodium vivax* malaria

8. A 45-year-old woman presents with pruritis, pale stools and dark urine. On examination she has finger clubbing and hepatospleno-megaly. Her blood tests reveal a normal bilirubin, elevated alkaline phosphatase and low T4. The MOST likely diagnosis is

A viral hepatitis
B chronic autoimmune active hepatitis
C suppurative cholangiohepatitis
D primary sclerosing cholangitis
E primary biliary cirrhosis

9. A 50-year-old man presents with a lump in the posterior triangle of the neck. It has been present for 8 months and is associated with a cheesy serous discharge. The MOST likely diagnosis is

A squamous cell carcinoma
B tuberculous adenitis
C deep lobe of parotid tumour
D infected branchial cyst
E sebaceous cyst

10) A 60-year-old African man presents with bone pain. His blood results are:

White cell count	3×10^9/L
Hb	9 g/dL with rouleaux formation
Platelets	70×10^9/L
ESR	120 mm/h
Plasma calcium	2.8 mmol/L
Alkaline phosphatase	100 IU/L (30–300 IU/L)
Creatinine	300 μmol/L
Urea	10 mmol/L

The MOST likely diagnosis is

A sickle cell disease
B multiple myeloma
C thrombotic thombocytopenic purpura
D polyarteritis nodosa
E primary hyperparathyroidism

11) A 22-year-old male presents with fever, sweating particularly at night, pruritus and weight loss. On examination he has palpable painless cervical lymph nodes and no skin manifestations. The MOST appropriate investigation would be

A full blood count
B lymph node biopsy
C chest x-ray
D CT scan of neck and mediastinum
E Mantoux test

12. A 70-year-old edentulous man presented with bruising and bone and joint pain. On examination he has nail splinters haemorrhages. The back of his legs are covered with haemorrhages into the muscles and ecchymoses. X-ray of his legs show subperiosteal haemorrhages. The MOST useful diagnostic text is

A capillary fragility test
B blood cultures
C bone marrow aspirate
D folic acid level
E platelet ascorbic acid levels

13. A 50-year-old renal transplant recipient on immunosuppressive therapy with ciclosporin, azathioprine and prednisolone is MOST at risk of developing

A squamous cell carcinoma of the skin
B basal cell carcinoma of the skin
C lymphoma
D liver failure
E leukaemia

14. A 17-year-old man with known sickle cell disease presents with severe lower back pain. He has a history of seizures. The FIRST step in management should be

A give oxygen at 4 L/min via a face mask
B start IV fluids
C give pethidine 150 mg IM every 2 hours until the pain settles
D give morphine 1–2 mg IV every 2–3 minutes until the pain settles
E lumbar spine and pelvic x-ray

15. A 40-year-old man with a prosthetic heart valve on warfarin anti-coagulation presents with haematuria. His INR is 4. The MOST appropriate management after withholding warfarin would be

A give 0.5–2 mg of vitamin K by slow IV injection
B no further treatment and recheck INR in 1–2 days
C commence heparin
D give 1 litre of FFP
E give prothrombin complex concentrate (Factor 9A) and Factor VII

16. Primary anti-phospholipid syndrome is associated with all of the following EXCEPT

A recurrent spontaneous abortion
B recurrent arterial thromboses
C recurrent venous thromboses
D thrombocytosis
E positive IgG anti-cardiolipin antibodies

17. Multiple myeloma is normally associated with all of the following EXCEPT

A β2-microglobulinuria
B high CRP
C high ESR
D urinary Bence Jones protein
E high paraprotein levels

18. The BEST drug treatment for refractory ventricular fibrillation is

A adrenaline (epinephrine)
B amiodarone
C lidocaine (lignocaine)
D adenosine
E esmolol

19. Which ONE of the following drugs may induce a psychosis similar to paranoid schizophrenia?

A heroin
B ecstasy (methylenedioxy methamfetamine)
C amphetamine
D cocaine
E barbiturates

20. A 25-year-old man presents to Casualty with repeated fits. He smells of alcohol and has jaw trismus. The MOST appropriate management is

A give 100 mg of IV thiamine
B give 50 ml of 50% glucose IV
C give 10 mg IV diazepam over 2 min.
D insert a Guedel oropharyngeal airway and prepare for endotracheal intubation
E insert a nasopharyngeal airway and administer oxygen

21. A 40-year-old man presents to Casualty within 1 hour of a paracetamol overdose. He smells of alcohol. His family confirms that he drinks heavily but is not on any medication. 16 tablets are missing from his paracetamol packs. The MOST appropriate management would be

A take emergency blood levels for paracetamol level
B give oral DL-methionine 2.5 g immediately followed by 50 mg of activated charcoal
C administer 50 mg of activated charcoal
D give IV N-acetylcysteine 150 mg/kg in 200 ml of 5% dextrose over 15 min.
E no treatment is required

22. A 55-year-old alcoholic is brought to Casualty by the police. He is confused and aggressive. There are no external signs of head trauma. Blood pressure is 140/90, heart rate 110 and he is pale. He has palmar erythema, tremors and smells of alcohol. The MOST important initial investigation for this man is

A blood alcohol level
B blood cultures
C gamma glutamyl transferase
D blood glucose
E clotting screen

23. His blood pressure drops to 100/60, and he begins to vomit. The MOST appropriate management would be

   A set up an IVI and give chlormethiazole infusion 0.8% (8 mg/ml), 40–80 ml over 10 minutes
   B give IM vitamin B complex
   C arrange urgent head CT scan and inform neurosurgeons
   D endotracheal intubation and gastric lavage
   E give 10 mg metoclopramide IV

24. Recognised side-effects of heparin include the following EXCEPT

   A thrombosis
   B thrombocytopenia
   C alopecia
   D osteoporosis
   E hypokalaemia

25. The following statements regarding statin lipid lowering drugs are correct EXCEPT

   A They should be initiated in patients with a coronary heart disease (CHD) risk >3% and with cholesterol concentrations >5 mmol/L.
   B They are advised for patients with triglyceride levels >5 mmol/L.
   C The upper age limit for initiating statin therapy for primary prevention is 69.
   D Pravastatin is the drug of choice for primary CHD prevention.
   E They act by inhibiting HMG CoA reductase.

26. The following statements regarding flecainide are correct EXCEPT

   A It blocks the inward sodium current in cardiac tissue.
   B It reduces automaticity.
   C It is safe in patients with heart failure.
   D It is a class I anti-arrhythmic drug.
   E It is used to terminate symptomatic acute atrial fibrillation of <48 hours.

27. A 50-year-old man complains of hardness of hearing and dyspnoea. He is noted to have a nasal septal perforation and a blood pressure of 140/90. His urinalysis shows red cells, protein and casts. The chest x-ray reveals opacities. The SINGLE investigation which is of greatest diagnostic value is

   A cytoplasmic anti-neutrophil cytoplasmic antibody (c-ANCA)
   B perinuclear (p-ANCA)
   C antinuclear antibody
   D antibasement membrane antibodies
   E Mantoux test

28. A 50-year-old woman presents with rheumatoid arthritis and weight loss. On examination she is noted to have splenomegaly and increased skin pigmentation. She has a positive rheumatoid factor. Her blood tests show neutropenia and normochromic normocytic anaemia. The MOST likely diagnosis is

A Sjögren's syndrome
B SLE
C amylordosis
D Felty's syndrome
E Caplan's syndrome

29. A 40-year-old woman complains of intolerance to cold weather and cold running water. On examination you note she has a beaked nose, radial furrowing of the lips and facial telangiectasiae. On examination of her hands you notice sausage-like digits and tapered fingers. The MOST likely diagnosis is

A SLE
B Sjögren's syndrome
C systemic sclerosis
D rheumatoid arthritis
E dermatomyositis

30. A 55-year-old man presents with an acutely painful swollen right knee. He recently was prescribed bendrofluazide for mild hypertension. The MOST useful investigation would be

A full blood count and ESR
B viral antibodies including parvovirus
C anti-nuclear antibody and rheumatoid factor
D aspirate of joint effusion for Gram stain and culture
E aspirate of joint effusion for polarised light microscopy

31. A 25-year-old man presents to Casualty with sudden onset of severe lower back pain that radiates down his right leg. On examination he is noted to have scoliosis of the spine, limited spinal flexion, restricted straight leg raise, limited hip movements and sensory loss over the dorsum of the right foot. The MOST likely diagnosis is

A spondylolisthesis
B ankylosing spondylitis
C acute cord compression
D lumbar canal stenosis
E lumbar disc prolapse

32. A 20-year-old woman presents with persistent cyanotic reticular mottling of the skin on the dorsum of her feet. The rash is accentuated in the cold. Temperature is 37.5°C, blood pressure 160/100, and trace proteinuria. Blood tests: elevated WBC with eosinophilia, normocytic normochromic anaemia and elevated ESR. The MOST likely diagnosis is

A Raynaud's phenomenon
B SLE
C polyarteritis nodosa
D rheumatoid arthritis
E Wegener's granulomatosis

33. The following auto-antibodies and diseases are correctly paired EXCEPT

A anti-striated muscle antibody – Dressler's syndrome
B anti-acetylcholine receptor antibody – myasthenia gravis
C anti-glomerular basement membrane antibody – Goodpasture's syndrome
D anti-intrinsic factor antibodies – pernicious anaemia
E p-ANCA – microscopic polyarteritis

34. The following statements regarding complement are correct EXCEPT

A Patients with hereditary angioedema have low levels of C1qEl.
B In Gram-negative sepsis, C3 is low and C4 is normal.
C C3 nephritis factor is associated with membrano-proliferative glomerulonephritis.
D SLE is associated with low C3 and normal C4.
E Hereditary angioedema is associated with normal C3 and low C4.

35. The MOST useful initial screening test for SLE is

A anti-dsDNA antibody
B anti-nuclear antibody
C anti-cardiolipin antibody
D C3 and C4 levels
E anti-extractable nuclear antigen (ENA) antibody

36. Rheumatoid arthritis may be associated with all of the following EXCEPT

A ulnar deviation
B carpal tunnel syndrome
C Dupuytren's contracture
D painful flexor tenosynovitis
E trigger finger

37. Cardinal signs of flexor tendon sheath infection include all of the following EXCEPT

A inability to move the digit
B tenderness over the flexor tendon sheath
C swelling
D slight flexion
E pain on passive extension of the digit

38. The diagnosis of acute recent myocardial ischaemia within minutes to 6 hours of the event is BEST confirmed by

A clinical history and examination
B presence of Q waves on 12-lead electrocardiogram
C presence of ST-segment elevation and T-wave inversion on 12-lead electrocardiogram
D elevated CK-MB enzymes
E elevated cardiac troponins I and T

39. A 60-year-old man presents with chest pain and sudden onset of atrial fibrillation with a heart rate of 160/min. The MOST appropriate management would be

A oxygen, heparin and synchronised DC shock
B oxygen, heparin, IV amiodarone
C oxygen, heparin, warfarin
D oxygen, beta-blockers
E oxygen, digoxin IV

40. Mitral regurgitation is BEST evaluated by

A M-mode echocardiogram
B 2D echocardiogram
C 12-lead electrocardiogram
D Doppler echocardiography
E thallium-201 nuclear scan

41. A 65-year-old man presents with an acute myocardial infarction with a new left bundle branch block. He had a haemorrhagic stroke a year ago. He is given 100% oxygen, diamorphine, metoclopramide, GTN and aspirin. The NEXT MOST appropriate management is

A IV glycoprotein IIb/ IIIa inhibitor
B thrombolytic therapy with streptokinase
C coronary artery bypass surgery
D percutaneous transluminal coronary angioplasty
E continuous infusion of heparin

42. A 50-year-old man presents with dyspnoea on exertion. On examination he has distended neck veins, hepatomegaly and ascites. He is also noted to have a paradoxical pulse and a rising JVP on inspiration. Chest x-ray reveals a small heart with calcification. The MOST likely diagnosis is

A viral pericarditis
B tuberculous pericarditis
C cardiac tamponade
D malignant pericarditis
E Dressler's syndrome

43. A 20-year-old woman presents with a BP of 170/100. She also complains of deteriorating vision and syncopal episodes. On examination she has impalpable peripheral pulses and systolic murmurs are auscultated above and below her clavicles. Her ESR is 50 mm/h. The MOST likely diagnosis is

A thrombangiitis obliterans
B coarctation of the aorta
C Kawasaki's disease
D Takayasu's disease
E Raynaud's disease

44. A 35-year-old IV drug abuser presents with right upper quadrant abdominal pain. On examination he has peripheral oedema, ascites and a tender liver. On chest auscultation he has a pansystolic murmur along the left sternal border. The MOST likely diagnosis is

A tricuspid regurgitation
B ventricular septal defect
C pulmonary stenosis
D mitral regurgitation
E atrial septal defect

45. A 60-year-old man in the Coronary Care Unit (CCU) has an elevated CVP reading a day after sustaining a myocardial infarction; this is confirmed on two further quarter hourly readings. On examination he has a few basal creps. He is asymptomatic. The MOST appropriate management would be

A give GTN, furosemide (frusemide) and an ACE inhibitor
B advise no added salt in diet
C give IV dopamine
D insert a Swan-Ganz catheter to assess LV filling pressures
E give 40 mg furosemide od

46. A 22-year-old woman presents with high blood pressure on routine physical examination. On examination she has a late systolic murmur and cold lower extremities. Her 12-lead ECG shows left ventricular hypertrophy. The MOST likely diagnosis is

A coarctation of the aorta
B systemic sclerosis
C Takayasu's arteritis
D Raynaud's disease
E SLE

47. The BEST investigation to diagnose a pulmonary embolism is

A arterial blood gases
B ventilation-perfusion isotope scintigraphy
C pulmonary angiogram
D 12-lead electrocardiogram
E PA and lateral chest x-ray

48. Which ONE of the following drugs is absolutely contraindicated in patients with asthma?

A adenosine
B atenolol
C adrenaline (epinephrine)
D verapamil
E bendrofluazide

49. A 60-year-old man has squamous cell carcinoma of the bronchus. The MOST useful investigation to assess curative surgical resection is

A radionucleotide scanning for the detection of metastatic disease
B fibreoptic bronchoscopy and cytology
C CT scan of the mediastinum
D measurement of FEV_1
E transthoracic fine-needle aspiration biopsy of mediastinal lymph node

50. A 20-year-old man presents with recurrent sinusitis and recurrent otitis media. On CT scan of the sinuses, the frontal sinuses are maldeveloped. On chest x-ray there are cystic shadows with fluid levels and dextrocardia. His 12-lead ECG shows inverted P-waves in lead I and reversed R wave progression. The MOST likely diagnosis is

A Down's syndrome
B Kartagener's syndrome
C Marfan's syndrome
D cystic fibrosis
E situs inversus

51. A 60-year-old man, with a history of COPD, presents to Casualty with a severe chest infection. On examination his temperature is 40°C, respiratory rate 32/minute, BP 120/55 and pulse rate is 110. Chest x-ray reveals a lobar pneumonia. He is not penicillin-allergic. The MOST appropriate therapy would be

A amoxicillin 500 mg o tds
B co-amoxyclavulanic acid 375 mg o tds + erythromycin 500 mg o qds
C cefotaxime 1–2 g IV tds + erythromycin 1g IV qds
D flucloxacillin 1–2 g IV qds + metronidazole 500 mg IV tds
E cefotaxime 1–2 g IV tds + gentamicin 2-5 mg/kg daily in 3 divided doses

52. Surgery for lung carcinoma is contraindicated in the presence of which ONE of the following?

A superior vena cava obstruction
B FEV_1 2 L
C tumour involving the first 1 cm of either main bronchus
D hypertrophic pulmonary osteoarthropathy
E haemoptysis

53. A 50-year-old man with lymphadenopathy confined to the mediastinum and pleural effusion is diagnosed as tuberculosis. He is HIV positive. The BEST management option would be

A 2 months of rifampicin, isoniazid, pyrazinamide and ethambutol then 4 months of rifampicin and isoniazid
B full regimen for 2 months then 10 months of rifampicin and isoniazid
C standard above TB therapy plus corticosteroids
D omit rifampicin and extend TB treatment to 18 months
E standard above TB therapy but reduce the dose of ethambutol

54. A 20-year-old woman is found unconscious. The results of her blood tests are as follows:

pH   7.2
plasma sodium   139 mmol/L
plasma potassium   4.2 mmol/L
plasma chloride   102 mmol/L
plasma HCO_3 11 mmol/L

These results are MOST compatible with

A aspirin poisoning
B meningitis
C Addison's disease
D hyperosmolar non-ketotic coma
E subarachnoid haemorrhage

55. A 45-year-old man presents with ptosis, meoisis and an unsteady gait. He is also noted to have bilateral gynaecomastia. The MOST likely diagnosis is

A alcoholism
B Klinefelter's syndrome
C heroin overdose
D Kallman's syndrome
E carcinoma of the lung

56. A 25-year-old man presents with weakness and numbness in his lower legs. He has just recovered from a recent chest infection. On examination deep tendon reflexes are absent and sensation is also lost. CSF from a lumbar puncture shows a normal cell count and glucose but raised protein level. The MOST likely diagnosis is

A mumps
B sarcoidosis
C AIDS
D Guillain–Barré syndrome
E Refsum's disease

57. The MOST useful step in guiding management would be

A pulse oximetry
B chest x-ray
C nerve conduction studies
D serial vital capacity
E serial peak flow measurement

58. A 50-year-old man presents with a sudden severe periorbital headache, neck pain and vomiting following sexual intercourse. The MOST useful investigation would be

A cerebral angiography
B carotid ultrasound and Doppler examination
C head CT scan
D full blood count and urea and electrolytes
E lumbar puncture

59. A 30-year-old man presents with a unilateral facial nerve palsy that involves his forehead. Possible causes include the following EXCEPT

A Bell's palsy
B Ramsay–Hunt syndrome
C acoustic neuroma
D cerebrovascular accident
E parotid tumour

60. Carpal tunnel syndrome is associated with all of the following EXCEPT

   A degenerative arthritis
   B pregnancy
   C acromegaly
   D Colles' fracture
   E diabetes

61. Claw hand deformity may be seen with all of the following EXCEPT

   A spinal cord injury
   B Charcot–Marie–Tooth disease
   C brachial plexus injuries
   D combined median and ulnar nerve lesion
   E rheumatoid arthritis

62. A 70-year-old man complains of flashing lights and floaters in his left eye for the past month and now complains of painless loss of vision in his left eye. The MOST likely diagnosis is

   A central retinal artery occlusion
   B central retinal vein occlusion
   C optic neuritis
   D retinal detachment
   E macular degeneration

63. A 30-year-old man presents with a right red painful eye. He complains of watering of the eyes and sensitivity to light. He has a history of recurrent cold sores. The MOST appropriate treatment is

   A prednisolone 0.5% 6 hourly
   B aciclovir 3% eye ointment 5 times daily
   C chloramphenicol 1% eye ointment
   D aciclovir 800 mg 5 times daily
   E cefuroxime 50 mg/ml

64. A 50-year-old woman presents with fever, headache, left eye pain and blurry vision. She states that she has just recovered from a cold. On examination she has a swollen left eyelid, mild proptosis and diminished visual acuity. She is unable to move her eye. The MOST likely diagnosis is

   A orbital cellulitis
   B giant-cell arteritis
   C sinusitis
   D choroiditis
   E cavernous sinus thrombosis

65. A 20-year-old man presents with a painful red eye. He has a long history of backache. On examination there is pus in the anterior chamber and synechiae. The MOST likely diagnosis is

A ankylosing spondylitis
B Reiter's syndrome
C Crohn's disease
D sarcoidosis
E rheumatoid arthritis

66. The following are possible responses to grief EXCEPT

A anger
B denial
C catatony
D guilt
E delirium

67. A 60-year-old woman presents with progressive forgetfulness and mood changes. She has a shuffling gait. Her brain CT scan shows cortical atrophy and enlarged ventricles. Histology shows senile plaques and neurofibrillary tangles. The MOST likely diagnosis is

A Wernicke–Korsakoff syndrome
B Parkinson's disease
C Alzheimer's disease
D variant Creutzfeldt–Jakob disease
E multi-infarct dementia

68. The following statements regarding venlafaxine are correct EXCEPT

A It has no affinity for adrenergic, cholinergic or histaminic receptors.
B It inhibits the reuptake of both serotonin and noradrenaline (norepinephrine).
C MAOIs may be taken in conjunction with venlafaxine.
D It is effective against chronic and refractory depression.
E Nausea is the MOST common side-effect.

69. The following statements regarding anorexia nervosa are true EXCEPT

A A BMI of <13 warrants hospital admission.
B Anorexia is defined as a BMI <17.5 associated with food avoidance.
C Physical features include bradycardia and hypotension.
D Investigations are important in confirming the diagnosis.
E Anorexia may be associated with reduced bone mass.

70. A 40-year-old man presents with dysphagia and epigastric pain not relieved by food and antacids. He has been taking NSAIDs for osteoarthritis of the hip for many months. On examination he has a palpable epigastric mass and a palpable supraclavicular lymph node. The MOST likely diagnosis is

A oesophageal squamous cell carcinoma
B duodenal ulcer
C peptic stricture of oesophagogastric junction
D gastric adenocarcinoma
E gastric ulcer

71. A 62-year-old man is admitted at 2AM with acute severe upper GI bleeding. On examination he is noted to have gynaecomastia and palmar erythema. His systolic BP is 90 and pulse 110. After starting him on IV gelofusin, ordering 6 units of blood and informing the duty surgeon, the NEXT MOST appropriate management would be

A emergency endoscopy
B sedate wth IV diazepam
C give stat dose of 50 μg IV octreotide followed by infusion at 50 μg/h
D insert gastroesophageal balloon to tamponade bleeding
E arrange endoscopy for the next routine list at 10 AM

72. A 25-year-old woman presents with 7 days of increasing bloody diarrhoea. She has just returned from Spain. On examination she has a temperature of 39°C and looks unwell. She is tender in the left lower quadrant of the abdomen. On proctoscopy it is difficult to see the mucosa, as it is obscured by blood and pus. The MOST appropriate management is

A send stool for microscopy and culture
B prescribe nightly hydrocortisone enema and oral mesalazine
C admit to hospital and ask GI surgeon to review
D prescribe tapering doses of oral prednisolone followed by olsalazine
E admit to hospital and arrange for urgent sigmoidoscopy and biopsies

73. A 50-year-old obese man presents complaining of recurrent abdominal pain radiating to the back and made worse by eating and bending over. Antacids relieve the pain. He smokes 20 cigarettes a day and drinks spirits daily. The MOST appropriate investigation would be

A oesophagogastroduodenoscopy
B double contrast barium meal
C Helicobacter pylori breath test
D abdominal ultrasound scan
E abdominal CT scan

74. The MOST likely diagnosis is

   A duodenal ulcer
   B gastro-oesophageal reflux disease (GORD)
   C acute pancreatitis
   D achalasia
   E Barrett's ulcer of the oesophagus

75. A 30-year-old man presents with cramping abdominal pain, diarr-hoea and weight loss. On examination: temperature 39°C; no lym-phadenopathy. Barium meal reveals a stricture in the terminal ileum. The MOST likely diagnosis is

   A tuberculosis
   B Crohn's disease
   C ulcerative colitis
   D lymphoma
   E coeliac disease

76. The BEST diagnostic test for Down's syndrome in a 10 week preg-nant woman is

   A triple blood test for serum oestriol, α-fetoprotein and β-human chorionic gonadotrophin
   B nuchal fold thickness scan
   C chorionic villus sampling
   D amniocentesis
   E chromosomal karyotyping of the parents

77. A 50-year-old man presents to Casualty with repeated fits. His plasma sodium is 112 mmol/L and urine osmolality is 550 mmol/kg. He is well hydrated. He smokes 20 cigarettes a day and drinks spir-its daily. The MOST likely diagnosis is

   A SIADH
   B Addison's disease
   C liver cirrhosis
   D renal failure
   E diabetes insipidus

78. The MOST appropriate treatment to correct his hyponatraemia is

   A desmopressin
   B terlipressin
   C demeclocycline
   D hydrocortisone
   E chlorthalidone

79. A 40-year-old obese man with non-insulin dependent diabetes takes metformin bd. His HbA1C returns as 13%. The MOST appropriate management would be

A commence insulin therapy
B increase metformin to tds and add repaglinide
C switch to gliclazide 40 mg daily
D continue current dose of metformin
E repeat HbA1C in a month's time and advise diet and exercise

80. A 60-year-old man presents to casualty drowsy and confused. Blood test results:

serum sodium	150 mmol/L
serum potassium	5 mmol/L
serum chloride	105 mmol/L
serum bicarbonate	30 mmol/L
serum urea	10 mmol/L
serum glucose	40 mmol/L

His serum osmolality is

A 260 mmol/L
B 280 mmol/L
C 300 mmol/L
D 340 mmol/L
E 360 mmol/L

81. A 40-year-old woman presents with a painful neck swelling. She had a chest infection a week prior. On examination: temperature is 39°C. The thyroid gland is diffusely enlarged and tender. T3 and T4 are both elevated but the radio-iodine uptake is decreased. The MOST likely diagnosis is

A Riedel's thyroiditis
B Grave's disease
C follicular thyroid carcinoma
D DeQuervain's thyroiditis
E Hashimoto's thyroiditis

82. On general examination a 48-year-old man referred to the Diabetic Clinic has coarse oily skin and a prominent supraorbital ridge. He has widely-spaced teeth and a moist handshake. The man's general appearance is MOST likely to be due to

A acromegaly
B haemochromatosis
C Klinefelter's syndrome
D gigantism
E thyrotoxicosis

83. The following statements regarding oral hypoglycaemic agents are true EXCEPT

A Chlopropamide is associated with facial flushing after alcohol ingestion.
B Gliblencamide is associated with risk of serious hypoglycaemia in patients >70.
C Repaglinide acts by inhibition of ATP-dependent potassium ion channels.
D Metformin is the drug of first choice in obese patients in whom strict dieting has failed.
E Tolbutamide is a biguanide.

84. A 30-year-old female presents with severe headache and vomiting. She is sensitive to light and also complains of neck pain. BP is 170/110 and pulse 50. On examination she has bilateral ptosis, dilated pupils and eyes are positioned down and out. On fundoscopy bilateral papilloedema is present. Protein and glucose are present in her urine.

The most appropriate investigation is

A lumbar puncture
B head CT scan
C MRI scan of the brain
D cerebral angiography
E electroencephalogram

85. In normal pregnancy which ONE of the following is true?

A The average weight gain is 20 kg.
B Haemoglobin levels rise.
C A progressive rise in plasma creatinine occurs.
D The cardiac output rises to term.
E The glomerular filtration rate and renal plasma flow rise by almost 50% by term.

86. Corticosteroid therapy reduces the progression towards renal failure in which ONE of the following conditions?

A post-streptococcal glomerulonephritis
B Berger's disease
C focal segmental glomerulosclerosis
D membranous glomerulonephritis
E rapidly progressive glomerulonephritis

87. You are called to see a 65-year-old woman with poor urine output. She is on IV flucloxacillin, benzylpenicillin and metronidazole for pelvic cellulitis. A Foley bladder catheter is inserted and the hourly urine output is confirmed as 10 ml/ hour. Her temperature is 38°C, blood pressure is 160/90 and pulse rate is 110. ECG shows peaked T waves and wide QRS complexes. Blood results include:

plasma sodium   139 mmol/L
plasma potassium   6.9 mmol/L
plasma urea   12 mmol/L
plasma creatinine   300 μmol/L

The MOST appropriate management for this patient is

A administer I litre of Hartmann's solution rapidly
B administer 20 ml of 10% calcium gluconate slowly into a central vein and administer 50 ml of 50% dextrose with 10 units of soluble human insulin over 30 min and thereafter at 10 ml/h
C administer 50–100 ml of 8.45% $NaHCO_3$ slowly IV into a central vein
D administer 120 mg furosemide (frusemide) as a bolus dose IV
E take blood cultures

88. The urine osmolality is 550 mosm/L, and urine sodium is 15 mmol/L. The MOST likely cause for her acute renal failure is

A acute tubular necrosis
B hypovolaemia
C sepsis
D acute interstitial nephritis
E rapidly progressive glomerulonephritis

89. A 30-year-old woman presents with fever, cough and haematuria. She had been in Egypt 2 weeks previously. On examination she has hepatomegaly. The drug treatment of CHOICE is

A hycanthone
B praziquantel
C quinine
D rifampicin, isoniazid, pyrazinamide and ethambutol
E sodium stibocaptate

90. A 50-year-old man presents with a red scaly rash over his neck and trunk, which has not responded to a 1-month course of topical corticosteroids. On examination he has randomly distributed serpiginous annular red plaques over his trunk and cervical lymphadenopathy. Blood test results are

white cell count	20×10^9/L with 50% eosinophils
Hb	10 g/dL
platelets	150×10^9/L

The MOST likely diagnosis is

A psoriasis
B mycosis fungoides
C solar keratosis
D pityriasis rosea
E lichen simplex

91. A 25-year-old man presents with non-pruritic white spots on his trunk. On examination there are multiple sharply demarcated round depigmented macules of up to 2 cm in size. On gentle scratching, a delicate scaling is noted. There is no associated lymphadenopathy. There is no family history of depigmentation. The MOST useful investigation is

A potassium hydroxide preparation of skin scrapings and direct microscopic examination
B skin smears for AFB
C syphilis serology
D full blood count and film
E HLA-B markers

92. A 50-year-old diabetic man presents with a necrolytic migratory erythematous rash. The MOST likely explanation for the rash is

A somatostatinoma
B vipoma
C glucagonoma
D insulinoma
E gastrinoma

93. A 60-year-old woman presents with a slowly-growing, painless but itchy flat red scaly plaque on her lateral lower calf. The MOST likely diagnosis is

A psoriasis
B granuloma annulare
C Bowen's disease
D squamous cell carcinoma
E necrobiosis lipoidica

94. A 50-year-old woman who is an avid sunbather presents with a red forehead with scaly rash. On examination, the lesions are multiple, discrete, small, erythematous, with a keratotic surface and varying from a few millimetres to up to 1 cm in diameter. The lesions are gritty to the touch. The MOST likely diagnosis is

A squamous cell carcinoma
B actinic keratosis
C discoid lupus erythematosus
D seborrheic keratosis
E psoriasis

95. She has tried topical diclofenac with no improvement. The next MOST appropriate treatment for this woman is

A curettage
B topical fluorouracil (Efudix)
C cryotherapy
D tangential excision
E photodynamic therapy

96. A 40-year-old man presents with a new intertriginous rash in both axillae. The area shows brown pigmentation in areas of multiple confluent papillomas. The rash is sometimes itchy. The MOST likely diagnosis for his rash is

A acanthosis nigricans
B dermatomyositis
C Addisonian hyperpigmentation
D porphyria cutanea tarda
E malignant melanoma

97. In the management of HIV in pregnancy, which ONE of the following drugs is CONTRAINDICATED?

A efavirenz
B lamivudine
C ritonavir
D zidovudine
E nelfinavir

98. Prophylaxis against opportunistic infections is advised when the CD4 count falls BELOW

A 500 cells/mm^3
B 300 cells/mm^3
C 250 cells/mm^3
D 200 cells/mm^3
E 100 cells/mm^3

99. All the following are opportunistic infections in HIV disease EXCEPT

A *Mycobacterium avium*
B *Toxoplasma gondii*
C *Pneumocystis carinii*
D cytomegalovirus
E *Helicobacter pylori*

100. A 20-year-old homosexual man presents with a greyish appearance at the lateral margins of the tongue. He does not drink or smoke and is not on any medication. The MOST likely infective cause is

A Epstein–Barr virus
B *Candida albicans*
C *Treponema pallidum*
D herpes simplex
E HIV

Answers to Paper Two BOFs

Criterion Referencing Marks

* *   – 25–50% of candidates expected to get correct
* ** – 50–75% of candidates expected to get correct
* *** – 75–100% of candidates expected to get correct

The notional PASS MARK is 72%

---

1. D *** This patient has oral candidiasis.

2. D ***

3. B *

4. A **

5. C **

6. A ***

7. C **

8. E ***

9. B ***

10. B **

11. B *** The patient has Hodgkin's disease.

12. E ***

13. A *

14. D * Seizures may be associated with pethidine.

15. C * Vitamin K may induce prolonged warfarin resistance in patients with prosthetic heart valves.

16. D ** Primary anti-phospholipid syndrome is associated with thrombocytopenia.

17. B ** Multiple myeloma is normally associated with low CRP. High CRP indicates concomitant infection.

18. B ***

19. C ***

20. E **

21. C **

22. D ***

23. A ***

24. E ** Heparin may be associated with hyperkalaemia and not hypokalaemia.

25. B ** They are advised for patients with a cholestrol level >5 mmol/L and increased coronary heart disease risk.

26. C ** Flecainide is contraindicated in the presence of heart failure.

27. A *** In Wegener's granulomatosis 90% will have an increase in cANCA and 20–40% will have elevated p-ANCA.

28. D ***

29. C ***

30. E ** This is a case of gout precipitated by thiazide diuretics.

31. E ***

32. C ** Livedo reticularis may be associated with PAN.

33. A *** Dressler's syndrome is associated with anti-cardiac muscle antibody.

34. D ** SLE is associated with low C3 and C4 levels.

35. B ***

36. C ***

37. A**

38. B ***

39. A **

40. D ***

41. D **

42. B ***

43. D ***

44. A *** The patient has infective endocarditis.

45. B **

46. A ***

47. C ***

48. B *** Beta-blockers and NSAIDs are contraindicated in patients with asthma.

49. C **

50. B **

51. C ** The patient has a severe community-acquired pneumonia.

52. A ***

53. D *

54. A ***

55. E ** Various neurological paraneoplastic syndromes, including cerebellar degeneration, are associated with small cell lung carcinoma.

56. D ***

57. D **

58. C *** Subarachnoid haemorrhage may present following sexual intercourse.

59. D ***

60. A ***

61. E **

62. D **

63. B **

64. A **

65. A ***

66. E ***

67. C ***

68. C * There should be a 14 day break between stopping MAOIs and commencing venlafaxine to avoid the serotonin syndrome.

69. D ***

70. D ***

71. A **

72. E **

73. A **

74. B ***

75. B ***

76. C *

77. A ***

78. C ***

79. B **

80. E *** The formula for calculating the serum osmolality = 2 (Na + K) + glucose + urea.

81. D **

82. A ***

83. E *** Tolbutamide is a sulfonylurea and metformin is a biguanide.

84. B ***

85. E *

86. D **

87. B ** The patient has prerenal failure.

88. C **

89. B ** Praziquantel available on named-patient basis for bilharzia.

90. B ***

91. A * The diagnosis is pityriasis versicolor alba.

92. C **

93. C **

94. B ***

95. B *

96. A *** Suspect carcinoma of the stomach.

97. A *

98. D **

99. E ***

100. A ***

MRCP Paper Three BOFs

In these questions candidates must select one answer only

Questions

1. A 40-year-old forester presents with a peculiar rash that started as a small papule. The rash now consists of multiple red rings up to 5 cm in diameter with raised borders and faded centres. He also complains of headache, fever and lymphadenopathy. The MOST likely diagnosis is

   A mycoplasma infection
   B *Borrelia burgdorferi* infection (Lyme disease)
   C tuberculosis
   D rheumatic fever
   E pityriasis rosea

2. Metronidazole is indicated for the treatment of all the following infections EXCEPT

   A bacterial vaginosis
   B trichomoniasis
   C *Giardia lamblia*
   D *Clostridium difficile*
   E *Chlamydia trachomatis*

3. A 22-year-old HIV-positive Ugandan man presents with hypopigmented anaesthetic annular lesions with raised erythematous rims and painful nodules on his left forearm and legs. On examination a thickened ulnar nerve is palpated at the left elbow and running into the lesions. He is also noted to have multiple transverse white lines on his fingernails. The MOST likely diagnosis is

   A leprosy
   B syphilis
   C leptospirosis
   D tuberculosis
   E sarcoidosis

4. A 45-year-old man presents with anorexia and weight loss. On examination he has a palpable, tender liver. Blood tests reveal a polymorph leucocytosis and a prolonged prothrombin time. The MCV is increased. The serum AST and ALT are only mildly elevated. The serum ferritin is 1000 μg/L. What is the definitive investigation for this man?

A CT scan of liver
B drug toxicology
C percutaneous or transjugular liver biopsy
D spiral CT scan of abdomen
E viral serology

5. A 40-year-old woman presents with dysuria and urinary incontinence. She has a history of having passed urinary calculi in the past. Her urine is noted to have an alkaline pH. The MOST likely organism is

A *Escherischia coli*
B *Proteus mirabilis*
C atypical streptococci
D *Pseudomonas aeruginosa*
E *Klebsiella* sp.

6. A 20-year-old HIV-positive man presents with fever and meningism. CSF shows:

pressure	250 mmH$_2$O
WBCs	200/mm^3
predom. cells	lymphocytes
glucose	33% plasma level
protein	5 g/L

Possible diagnoses include the following EXCEPT

A cryptococcal meningitis
B coccidioides meningitis
C tuberculous meningitis
D carcinomatous meningitis
E histoplasma meningitis

7. The following statements regarding human parvovirus B19 are correct EXCEPT

A may cause aplastic crises in patients with sickle cell disease
B produces erythema infectiosum
C produces hand foot and mouth disease
D causes chronic anaemia in immunocompromised patients
E may cause aplastic crises in patients with hereditary spherocytosis

8. A 70-year-old man, who lives alone and is self-caring, presents with weakness in his lower legs and muscle pain. On examination he has loose teeth and is noted to have ecchymoses of the lower limbs. He suffers from rheumatoid arthritis, which greatly limits his mobility. The MOST likely diagnosis is

A folate deficiency
B scurvy
C iron deficiency
D thiamine deficiency
E vitamin B$_{12}$ deficiency

9. A 35-year-old African woman is found to have a Hb of 6 g/dL. She is a vegetarian and has a history of uterine fibroids. Her blood film reveals microcytic, hypochromic red blood cells and a few target cells. The MOST likely diagnosis is

A thalassaemia trait
B iron-deficiency anaemia
C sickle cell disease
D anaemia of chronic disease
E sideroblastic anaemia

10. A 25-year-old woman presents with a single, non-tender enlarged cervical lymph node. She also complains of fever and night sweats. Lymph node biopsy reveals infiltration with histiocytes and lymphocytes and the presence of cells with bi-lobed mirror-image nuclei. The MOST likely diagnosis is

A non-Hodgkin's lymphoma
B Hodgkin's lymphoma
C sarcoidosis
D acute lymphoblastic leukaemia
E tuberculosis

11. A 22-year-old male presents with fever, sweating particularly at night, pruritus and weight loss. On examination he has palpable painless cervical lymph nodes and no skin manifestations. The MOST likely diagnosis is

A tuberculosis
B non-Hodgkin's lymphoma
C Hodgkin's lymphoma
D acute lymphoblastic leukaemia
E chronic lymphocytic leukaemia

12. The following statements regarding amiodarone are correct EXCEPT

    A Amiodarone is a class Ib anti-arrhythmic drug.
    B It acts to prolong the action potential.
    C It does not affect sodium transport through the membrane.
    D It is arrhythmogenic if given with drugs that prolong the QT interval.
    E It is associated with abnormalities of thyroid function.

13. The absolute contraindication to thrombolytic therapy IS

    A INR >2.5
    B recent head trauma
    C suspected aortic dissection
    D known bleeding disorder
    E pregnancy

14. Which one of the following drugs CANNOT be administered via the tracheal route?

    A adrenaline (epinephrine)
    B atropine
    C amiodarone
    D lidocaine (lignocaine)
    E naloxone

15. The following cardiac drugs are correctly paired with their corresponding indications for use EXCEPT

    A amiodarone – haemodynamically stable ventricular tachycardia
    B lidocaine (lignocaine) – first-line drug for refractory ventricular fibrillation
    C magnesium sulphate – torsades de pointes
    D adenosine – paroxysmal supraventricular tachycardia
    E verapamil – supraventricular tachycardia

16. The following statements regarding digoxin are true EXCEPT

    A It increases vagal tone.
    B It decreases sympathetic drive.
    C It increases conduction velocity in the Purkinje fibres.
    D It is less effective than amiodarone in acute atrial fibrillation.
    E It prolongs AV node refractory period.

17. The following statements regarding tricyclic antidepressant poisoning are correct EXCEPT

A It may be treated by activated charcoal.
B Oral diazepam is usually adequate to sedate delirious patients.
C The use of anti-arrhythmics is strongly advised.
D It is associated with dilated pupils and urinary retention.
E It is associated with hypothermia and hyper-reflexia.

18. Recommended treatment for salicylate poisoning includes all of the following EXCEPT

A forced alkaline diuresis
B haemodialysis
C activated charcoal by mouth
D urinary alkalinisation with sodium bicarbonate
E charcoal haemoperfusion

19. A 60-year-old woman presents with progressive forgetfulness and mood changes. She has a shuffling gait. Her brain CT scan shows cortical atrophy and enlarged ventricles. Histology shows senile plaques and neurofibrillary tangles. The MOST appropriate treatment is

A levodopa in combination with a dopa-decarboxylase inhibitor
B donepezil
C tetrabenazine
D diazepam
E thiamine

20. The following statements regarding anti-epileptic drugs are correct EXCEPT

A Carbamazepine is the drug of choice for absence seizures.
B Sodium valproate is the drug of choice for myoclonic seizures.
C Lamotrigine is the drug of choice for seizures associated with Lennox–Gastaut syndrome.
D Carbamazepine may be used as prophylaxis of bipolar disorder unresponsive to lithium.
E Carbamazepine is associated with Stevens–Johnson syndrome.

21. A 50-year-old man complains of difficulty in hearing and dyspnoea. He is noted to have a nasal septal perforation and a blood pressure of 140/90. His urinalysis shows red cells, protein and casts. The chest x-ray reveals opacities. The MOST appropriate treatment for the condition described is

   A rifampicin, isoniazid, pyrazinamide and ethambutol
   B cyclophosphamide
   C plasmaphoresis
   D penicillin
   E short-course of prednisolone

22. The following clinical manifestations are associated with sarcoidosis EXCEPT

   A finger clubbing
   B lupus pernio
   C pulmonary fibrosis
   D erythema nodosum
   E facial nerve palsy

23. A 40-year-old man presents with a painful and swollen right knee joint. The synovial fluid is opaque and bloody with no white cells or crystals. Possible diagnoses include the following EXCEPT

   A Charcot joint
   B haemophilia
   C osteosarcoma
   D aseptic necrosis
   E chondrocalcinosis

24. A 40-year-old woman complains of difficulty placing an object on a high shelf and of combing her hair. She also has trouble climbing and descending the stairs. She adds that she has difficulty swallowing food. She is sensitive to the cold and does not smoke or drink alcohol. On examination, she has weakness in the muscles of the neck, shoulder girdle, hips and thighs. Deep tendon reflexes are mildly reduced. Her blood tests reveal elevated creatinine kinase, AST, ALT and LDH. Electromyography shows fibrillation potentials. The MOST likely diagnosis is

   A Eaton–Lambert syndrome
   B amyotophic lateral sclerosis
   C dystrophia myotonica
   D polymyositis
   E myasthenia gravis

25. A 60-year-old woman presents with morning stiffness in both knees and pain worse at the end of the day. On examination the knees are swollen and warm to the touch with a flexion deformity and limitation of movement. X-ray shows narrowing of the joint spaces, osteophytes at the margin of the joints and sclerosis of the underlying bone. The MOST likely diagnosis is

A rheumatoid arthritis
B osteoarthritis
C gout
D infective arthritis
E polymyalgia rheumatica

26. A 20-year-old pregnant black woman presents with fever and joint pains. She has a history of two previous spontaneous early miscarriages. Her urine reveals 2+ protein. Her blood results show leucopenia, normocytic normochromic anaemia and thrombocytopenia. The MOST sensitive diagnostic test would be

A positron emission tomography (PET scan)
B antibodies to double-stranded DNA
C anti-nuclear antibodies
D antibody to Ro
E haemoglobin electrophoresis

27. The following statements regarding acute myocardial infarction are correct EXCEPT

A A lateral infarction is usually seen in leads V5–6 and/or leads I and aVL.
B An inferior infarction results often from a lesion in the right coronary artery.
C Patients with an anterior infarction benefit more from thrombolysis and treatment with ACE inhibitors than at other sites.
D Acute coronary syndrome is defined as infarction with new LBBB.
E Initial management for acute MI should include morphine, oxygen, GTN and aspirin.

28. The following statements regarding electrocardiography are correct EXCEPT

A Electrodes should be placed over muscle not bone to minimise electrical interference.
B A completely straight line usually does not indicate asystole.
C Standard paper speed is 25 mm/s.
D Pulseless electrical activity signifies the absence of cardiac output in the presence of any form of electrical activity.
E Fine ventricular fibrillation (VF) has a worse prognosis than coarse VF.

29. The following statements regarding the internal jugular vein (IJV) are correct EXCEPT

A It initially lies in front of the carotid artery.
B As it descends in the neck it lies lateral to the common carotid artery.
C On the right it joins the subclavian vein to form the brachiocephalic vein.
D IX–XII cranial nerves and the phrenic nerve are closely related to the IJV in the neck.
E The site of insertion for central vein cannulation is the apex of the triangle formed by the two heads of the sternomastoid muscle.

30. A 50-year-old man presents with bradycardia of 30 beats/min. His systolic blood pressure is 80. He has a productive pink frothy cough and basal crackles on auscultation. ECG confirms sinus bradycardia and inferior myocardial infarction. There has been no satisfactory response to an initial 500 µg IV of atropine. The NEXT most appropriate management for this man would be

A repeat atropine to maximum 3 mg
B adrenaline (epinephrine) 2–10 µg/min as an IV bolus
C isoprenaline IV infusion
D transcutaneous pacing on the T wave
E transvenous pacing

31. A 70-year-old man presents to the outpatient clinic with a 2-month history of worsening breathlessness and chest pain on exertion. On examination you note an ejection systolic murmur in the aortic region, an early high-pitched diastolic murmur at the left lower sternal edge and pulsus biferiens. The MOST likely diagnosis is

A infective endocarditis
B left atrial myxoma
C rheumatic aortic valvular disease
D impending myocardial infarction
E congestive cardiac failure

32. The MOST useful investigation would be

A 12-lead electrocardiogram
B echocardiogram
C cardiac catheterisation
D cardiac isoenzymes and troponin
E chest x-ray

33. A 55-year-old smoker with a history of chronic productive cough presents to Casualty breathless and drowsy. On examination he is centrally cyanosed with a raised JVP and a palpable liver. There is a pansystolic murmur at the lower left sternal border. No abnormality is heard in the lungs. The MOST likely diagnosis is

A infective endocarditis
B cor pulmonale
C ventricular septal defect
D exacerbation of chronic bronchitis
E emphysema

34. The MOST useful diagnostic investigation is

A arterial blood gas
B 12-lead electrocardiogram
C lung function tests
D chest x-ray
E blood cultures

35. The MOST appropriate treatment is

A continuous oxygen therapy
B furosemide (frusemide)
C salbutamol inhaler
D oral prednisolone 30 mg od
E amoxicillin 500 mg o tds

36. The inspired oxygen content using a bag-valve-mask with oxygen but no reservoir is

A 16%
B 21%
C 40%
D 50%
E 85%

37. The following are recognised features of obstructive sleep apnoea (OSA) EXCEPT

A hypnagogic hallucinations
B impotence
C morning headaches
D nightmares
E daydreaming

38. A 20-year-old arrives to Casualty with marked dyspnoea; he suffers from asthma. On examination respiratory rate 24/min and pulse 105/min. The peak flow is 60% of predicted. The MOST appropriate management would be

A Treat in casualty with nebulised salbutamol 5 mg and repeat peak flow in 30 min.
B Arrange immediate hospital admission and treat with IV hydrocortisone 200 mg.
C Arrange immediate hospital admission, administer oxygen 40–60%, nebulised salbutamol and oral prednisolone 30–60 mg.
D Arrange immediate hospital admission, administer oxygen-driven nebuliser and give slow IV aminophyline 250 mg.
E Treat in casualty with oral prednisolone 30–60 mg and repeat peak flow in 30 min.

39. An 18-year-old man presents with fever, stridor and trismus. His breathing becomes laboured with use of accessory muscles. He becomes cyanosed with a respiratory rate of 35, despite oxygen by face mask. He had initially presented to his GP a few days ago with a sore throat. He takes salbutamol inhaler for his asthma. The MOST appropriate management in Casualty would be

A endotracheal intubation
B needle cricothyroidotomy
C tracheostomy
D IV hydrocortisone
E nasopharyngeal airway

40. The MOST likely diagnosis is

A glandular fever
B streptococcal throat infection
C acute asthma attack
D angioneurotic oedema
E tetanus

41. A 60-year-old priest presents with cough, dyspnoea, dull chest pain and vague epigastric pain. On examination the left chest shows diminished expansion, stony dull percussion note and absent breath sounds. There is aegophony at the apex. The mediastinum is shifted to the right. The chest x-ray confirms a unilateral pleural effusion. The MOST useful investigation would be

A CT chest
B sputum for culture and sensitivity
C aspiration of pleural effusion
D bronchoscopy
E V/Q scan

42. A 60-year-old dairy farmer presents with fever, cough and shortness of breath. Coarse end-inspiratory crackles are present. Chest x-ray shows bilateral fluffy nodular shadows. The MOST likely diagnosis is

A extrinsic allergic alveolitis
B aspergilloma
C cryptogenic fibrosing alveolitis
D histoplasmosis
E blastomycosis

43. Examples of physiological shunting include all of the following EXCEPT

A pulmonary fibrosis
B pulmonary embolism
C pulmonary oedema
D COPD
E atelectasis

44. A 30-year-old female involved in a road traffic accident is brought by ambulance to Casualty. She is noted to have bruising over the mastoid process and periorbital haematoma. On otoscopic examination she has bleeding behind the tympanic membrane. The MOST likely diagnosis is

A extradural haematoma
B subdural haematoma
C basal skull fracture
D depressed occipital skull fracture
E intracerebral haemorrhage

45. A 60-year-old man presents with rigidity and bradykinesia. He has an ataxic gait. On examination he has postural hypotension without compensatory tachycardia and his pupils are asymmetric. The MOST likely diagnosis is

A multi-infarct dementia
B Alzheimer's disease
C Friedreich's ataxia
D Parkinson's disease
E Shy–Drager syndrome

46. The following pathological findings and diseases are correctly paired EXCEPT

A Lewy bodies – Parkinson's disease
B plaques of demyelination – multiple sclerosis
C neurofibrillary tangles – Alzheimer's disease
D Negri bodies – rabies
E sulphur granules – variant CJD (related to BSE)

47. A 40-year-old man is brought to Casualty in a comatose state. Useful initial investigations include all of the following EXCEPT

  A serum glucose
  B serum calcium
  C arterial blood gases
  D full blood count
  E blood alcohol level

48. On examination he is noted to have constricted pupils and depressed respirations. The MOST appropriate management would be:

  A head CT scan
  B naloxone 0.4–1.2 mg IV stat
  C flumazenil 200 mcg IV over 15 s
  D doxapram IV
  E dantrolene 1 mg/kg IV

49. A 20-year-old man is found unconscious after a night of binge drinking. There is no evidence of physical trauma. On examination he has alcohol on his breath and a bitten tongue. Blood pressure 110/80 and pulse 80/min. The pupils are small, equal and responsive to light. On removal of his clothes, his trousers are noted to be soiled with urine. The MOST likely explanation for his unconscious state is

  A hypoglycaemic coma
  B alcoholic overdose
  C post-ictal phase of an epileptic seizure
  D subarachnoid haemorrhage
  E narcotic drug overdose

50. A 40-year-old pedestrian has been struck by a speeding car. He is brought to Casualty wearing a pneumatic antishock garment for an extensive open avulsion injury to his pelvis. He is intubated with fluids running via two large-bore intravenous cannulas. His blood pressure is 120/80. The pelvis is grossly distorted. The NEXT most appropriate management as a casualty officer would be

  A take blood for full blood count, type and cross 6 units, urea and electrolytes and commence O negative blood infusion
  B cut away the man's clothing and perform a thorough physical examination
  C insert a Foley catheter after a digital rectal examination to exclude a high riding prostate
  D perform a brief neurological examination
  E notify the orthopaedic surgeons to apply an external fixator

51. A 25-year-old man presents with unilateral eye pain of acute onset, blurring of vision, photophobia, lacrimation, red eye and a small pupil. The pain is exacerbated on testing of accommodation and the pupil is seen to constrict. The MOST likely diagnosis is

A acute closed angle glaucoma
B acute iritis
C acute conjunctivitis
D ulcerative keratitis
E subconjunctival haemorrhage

52. A 40-year-old man presents with dry cough, exertional dyspnoea and weight loss. On examination he is noted to have finger clubbing and fine end-inspiratory crepitations are heard. Chest x-ray shows bilateral reticulonodular shadowing at the lung bases. Lung function tests show reduced lung volumes, normal FEV_1 and FVC ratio but reduced individual values, and reduced transfer factor. ANA and rheumatoid factor are absent. The MOST likely diagnosis is

A extrinsic allergic alveolitis
B sarcoidosis
C lymphangiitis carcinomatosa
D cryptogenic fibrosing alveolitis
E histiocytosis X

53. A 20-year-old man presents with persistent eye irritation. He explains that he is sensitive to light, has noted worsening vision and complains of aching eyes. He also complains of morning stiffness in his back. The MOST likely diagnosis is

A keratitis
B uveitis
C viral conjunctivitis
D episcleritis
E choroiditis

54. The MOST useful investigation for this man would be

A lumbar and pelvic spine x-ray
B Kveim test
C HIV test
D Mantoux test
E rheumatoid factor

55. A 70-year-old long-sighted woman presents to Casualty at midnight with vomiting that began three hours earlier and slightly worsening vision. The eyeball is rock-hard on palpation. The conjunctiva is injected. The MOST appropriate management for this patient is

A dilate pupil with tropicamide to examine the retina
B give antiemetic and refer to ophthamologist in the morning
C oral prednisolone
D give antiemetic and IV acetazolamide (diamox) and refer to on-call ophthalmologist urgently
E prescribe fucithalmic ointment bd

56. The following statements regarding Good Medical Practice (GMC code) are correct EXCEPT

A You must provide the necessary care to alleviate pain and distress whether or not curative treatment is possible.
B You may end a professional relationship with a patient if he or she makes a complaint about you or your team.
C In an emergency, wherever it may arise, you must offer anyone at risk the assistance you could reasonably be expected to provide.
D You must respond constructively to the outcome of appraisals of your performance.
E You must take part in adverse event recognition and reporting to help reduce risk to patients.

57. Diagnostic features of post-traumatic stress disorder include all of the following EXCEPT

A autonomic arousal
B recurrent, obtrusive thoughts
C symptoms of anxiety
D memory impairment
E loss of orientation

58. Diagnostic features of panic disorder include all of the following EXCEPT

A dizziness
B feelings of unreality
C fear of insanity
D fear of leaving home
E choking sensations

59. Diagnostic features of mania include all of the following EXCEPT

A labile mood
B rapid speech
C loss of inhibitions
D overeating
E grandiosity

60. The following statements regarding Good Medical Practice are correct EXCEPT

A You may end professional relationships with patients if they have persistently acted inconsiderately.
B You must assist the coroner by offering all relevant information to an inquest.
C You are not entitled to remain silent if your evidence may lead to criminal proceedings being taken against you.
D If you have grounds to believe that a doctor may be putting patients at risk, you must give an honest explanation of your concerns to a medical director.
E You must not refuse to treat a patient because you may be putting yourself at risk.

61. A 45-year-old woman presents with pruritis, pale stools and dark urine. On examination she has finger clubbing and hepatospleno-megaly. Her blood tests reveal a normal bilirubin, elevated alkaline phosphatase and low T4. The MOST certain way to confirm the diagnosis is by

A anti-mitochondrial antibody
B liver biopsy
C ERCP
D CT scan of the abdomen
E hepatitis A, B and C serology

62. A 22-year-old woman, back from Thailand a fortnight ago, is rushed to casualty in a comatose state. On examination she is jaundiced and unrousable. Her reflexes are exaggerated. The MOST appropriate treatment for this patient is

A give quinine dihydrochloride 10–20 mg/kg loading dose then 10 mg/kg 8 hourly IV
B administer IV fluids and supportive therapy
C give mefloquine in a stat dose of 15 mg/kg then 10 mg/kg 8 hours later
D give chloroquine
E give suramin 200 mg IV test dose and then 20 mg/kg IV on 5–10 occasions at 5-day intervals and add malarsoprol on day 8

63. A 60-year-old man presents with increasing abdominal girth. On examination you elicit shifting dullness. The MOST useful investigation would be

A CT scan of the abdomen
B ascitic fluid tap
C ultrasound of the abdomen
D chest x-ray
E blood for FBC, urea and electrolytes, LFTs and amylase

64. A 65-year-old man presents with a 2-month history of vague lower abdominal pain, alternating diarrhoea and constipation and 4-kg weight loss. He has passed a small amount of dark red blood per rectum. He is anaemic. The MOST useful investigation is

A flexible sigmoidoscopy
B barium enema
C CT scan of abdomen
D abdominal ultrasound
E selective mesenteric angiography

65. A 50-year-old woman presents to medical outpatients complaining of pain and stiffness in the joints of her hands, worse in the mornings. The pain lasts for a couple of hours in the morning. On examination she has ulnar deviation, wasting of the small muscles of her hands, nail pitting and a rash on her knees. There is symmetrical involvement of the distal interphalangeal joints and metacarpophalangeal joints. The MOST likely diagnosis is

A rheumatoid arthritis
B psoriatic arthropathy
C dermatomyositis
D SLE
E osteoarthritis

66. Causes of air under the diaphragm include all of the following EXCEPT

A Crohn's disease
B perforated duodenal ulcer
C pleuroperitoneal fistula
D laparoscopy
E ruptured ectopic pregnancy

67. A 50-year-old man presents in shock with rigors and a temperature of 40°C. He is jaundiced and is tender on palpation of the liver, which is felt 5 cm below the costal margin. Dark concentrated urine is noted upon Foley catheter insertion. The MOST likely diagnosis is

A ascending cholangitis
B gallstone ileus
C hepatitis
D primary sclerosing cholangitis
E acute cholecystitis

68. A 54-year-old diabetic man presents with fever, and a painful and swollen right lower leg. On examination, the pulses are absent distally, the foot cold and subcutaneous crepitus is present. The MOST useful investigation is

A x-ray of the leg
B Doppler ultrasound
C arteriogram
D blood cultures
E venogram

69. The MOST likely diagnosis is

A osteomyelitis
B gas gangrene
C chronic ischaemia of the leg
D deep venous thrombosis
E acute ischaemia of the leg

70. A 66-year-old woman presents in a coma. Temperature 35°C, pulse 50 and BP 140/80. On examination she has a goitre and few basal rales in the chest. Her medication is thyroxine, bendrofluazide, and omeprazole. Blood results:

plasma sodium	129 mmol/L
plasma potassium	3.6 mmol/L
plasma urea	10 mmol/L
plasma creatinine	130 µmol/L
plasma glucose	3 mmol/L

The MOST likely underlying diagnosis is

A renal failure
B Addisonian crisis
C hypoglycaemia
D congestive heart failure
E myxoedema

71. A 55-year-old man complains of generalised weakness for the past month. He also complains of excessive thirst and frequent micturition. Blood results:

urine glucose	negative
urine nitrate	negative
serum creatinine	140 µmol/L
serum urea	10 mmol/L
serum calcium	3.5 mmol/L
serum phosphate	1 mmol/L
serum alkaline phosphatase	200 IU/L (30–300 IU/L)
serum albumin	45 g/L

These findings are consistent with all of the following diseases EXCEPT

A primary hyperparathyroidism
B sarcoidosis
C multiple myeloma
D thyrotoxicosis
E bone metastases

72. The following are useful investigations to establish the diagnosis EXCEPT

A full blood count
B chest x-ray
C ESR
D parathyroid hormone
E magnesium

73. A 65-year-old man presents with a 2-month history of vague lower abdominal pain, alternating diarrhoea with constipation and 4 kg weight loss. He has passed a small amount of dark red blood per rectum. There is anaemia. The MOST likely diagnosis is

A diverticular disease
B Crohn's disease
C ulcerative colitis
D angiodysplasia
E colorectal cancer

74. A 25-year-old woman presents to the outpatient clinic with a neck swelling. On examination the swelling moves upward with protrusion of the tongue. The MOST likely diagnosis is

A thyroid goitre
B cystic hygroma
C thyroglossal cyst
D branchial cyst
E thyroid malignancy

Paper Three BOFs questions

75. The following are recognised causes of respiratory alkalosis
EXCEPT

A high altitude
B salicylates
C pulmonary emboli
D right to left pulmonary shunt
E flail chest

76. The following are recognised causes of mixed metabolic alkalosis
and respiratory alkalosis EXCEPT

A pregnancy and vomiting
B hepatic failure and diuretics
C chronic respiratory failure and mechanical ventilation
D Gram-negative septicaemia
E massive blood transfusion

77. Causes of hypercalcaemia associated with decreased parathyroid
hormone include all of the following EXCEPT

A Addison's disease
B thyrotoxicosis
C recovery from acute tubular necrosis
D Paget's disease
E immobilisation

78. The BEST initial investigation of female infertility is

A transvaginal ultrasound
B chromosomal karyotype
C prolactin level
D demonstration of rise of progesterone during the luteal phase
E diagnostic laparoscopy

79. A 20-year-old woman presents with secondary amenorrhoea. The
urine pregnancy test is negative. Her basal plasma prolactin level is
350 mU/L (60–390). She is given a progestogen challenge and has
withdrawal bleeding. The MOST likely diagnosis is:

A polycystic ovarian disease
B prolactinoma
C gonadal dysgenesis
D chronic anovulation with oestrogen absent
E Mullerian agenesis

80. Causes of hyperprolactinaemia include all of the following EXCEPT

A hyperthyroidism
B sarcoidosis
C metoclopramide
D pituitary tumour
E pregnancy

81. The following statements regarding parathyroid hormone (PTH) are correct EXCEPT

A Pseudohypoparathyroidism is due to failure of target cells to respond to PTH.
B Secondary hyperparathyroidism is associated with raised PTH appropriate to low calcium.
C Secondary hyperparathyroidism usually occurs following neck surgery.
D The most common cause of primary hyperparathyroidism is a single benign adenoma.
E Primary hyperparathyroidism is associated with MEN type I.

82. A 60-year-old man presents to Casualty with painless profuse haematuria for the past 2 days. On examination BP 90/50 and pulse 105/min. Blood results:

white cell count	5×10^9/L
Hb	6 g/dL
platelets	150×10^9/L
serum creatinine	300 μmol/L
serum urea	20 mmol/L

Following resuscitation, the patient is no longer bleeding. The MOST useful investigation would be

A cystoscopy
B intravenous pyelogram
C ultrasound of the kidneys, bladder and prostate
D pelvic CT scan
E retrograde urography

83. A 42-year-old woman presents to Casualty with right-sided colicky loin pain and nausea for the past 3 hours. She cannot keep still because of the pain. She has a history of recurrent cystitis. Temperature 36.5°C, BP 110/60 and pulse 60/min. Urinalysis shows microscopic haematuria. The MOST likely diagnosis is

A pelvic inflammatory disease
B acute pyelonephritis
C acute appendicitis
D nephrolithiasis
E ectopic pregnancy

84. The MOST useful initial diagnostic investigation is

A serum urea and electrolytes
B urine β-HCG
C plain KUB film
D pelvic ultrasound
E IV urogram

85. A 16-year-old male presents with gynaecomastia. On examination his arm span exceeds the trunk length and he has small, firm testes. The following conditions are associated with short stature EXCEPT

A achondroplasia
B hypopituitarism
C rickets
D Crohn's disease
E Klinefelter's syndrome

86. A 70-year-old man presents to the outpatient clinic complaining of difficulty urinating and dribbling. On abdominal examination he has a distended bladder that reaches the umbilicus. He also complains of back pain. The NEXT most appropriate step would be

A take blood for serum urea, creatinine and electrolytes
B take blood for PSA and acid phosphatase
C perform a digital rectal examination
D insert a Foley catheter
E MSU for urinalysis and MC&S

87. Causes of proximal renal tubular acidosis include all of the following EXCEPT

A Wilson's disease
B carbonic anhydrase inhibitors
C multiple myeloma
D hyperparathyroidism
E chronic active hepatitis

88. A 40-year-old man presents with fever, backache and acute obstructive renal failure. Hb is 9 g/dL, and he has a raised ESR. IV urogram shows dilated ureters with medial deviation of the ureters. The MOST likely diagnosis is

A ureteric stone obstruction
B obstructive megaureter
C retroperitoneal fibrosis
D pelvi-ureteric junction obstruction
E obstructive nephropathy secondary to malignancy

89. A 30-year-old woman with Crohn's disease presents with left flank pain and microscopic haematuria. She admits she doesn't drink enough water. She smokes, drinks wine and loves chocolates. X-ray shows a radiopaque left renal calculus. The MOST likely aetiology is

A hypercalciuria
B hyperoxaluria
C hyperuricaemia
D cystinuria
E hyperuricosuria

90. A 30-year-old man presents with fever and jaundice. He enjoys travelling and water sports and has recently returned from Sri Lanka. On examination he is also noted to have injected conjunctivae and hepatomegaly. His Hb is low, and he has microscopic haematuria. ESR, serum creatinine and urea are markedly raised, and his serum transaminases are only slightly raised. The treatment of choice is

A metronidazole
B penicillin
C ciprofloxacin
D tetracycline
E doxycycline

91. A 25-year-old man presents with non-pruritic white spots on his trunk. On examination there are multiple sharply demarcated round depigmented macules of up to 2 cm in size. On gentle scratching, a delicate scaling is noted. There is no associated lymphadenopathy. There is no family history of depigmentation. Organisms are seen on direct microscopy. The MOST likely diagnosis is

A psoriasis
B pinta
C leprosy
D vitiligo
E pityriasis versicolor alba

92. White nails are associated with all of the following conditions EXCEPT

A psoriasis
B renal failure
C arsenic poisoning
D cytotoxic drug therapy
E cirrhosis

93. A 45-year-old woman with diabetes presents with shiny waxy erythematous plaques on her shins with yellowish skin and telangiectasia. The MOST likely diagnosis is

A pretibial myxoedema
B pyoderma gangrenosum
C psoriasis
D erythema nodosum
E necrobiosis lipoidica

94. A 30-year-old man presents with fever, arthralgia and a palmar rash. On examination he has oral vesicles and circular lesions on his palms. The MOST likely diagnosis is

A Stevens–Johnson syndrome
B Behçet's syndrome
C herpes simplex
D syphilis
E hand-foot-mouth disease

95. Photodermatitis is a complication of all of the following drugs EXCEPT

A demeclocycline
B furosemide (frusemide)
C oral contraceptives
D nalidixic acid
E barbiturates

96. Alopecia is a recognised complication of all of the following EXCEPT

A withdrawal from oral contraceptives
B heparin
C ethionamide
D cytotoxic drugs
E sulfonamides

97. A 16-year-old girl is brought to Casualty by her mother. She complains of persistent and worsening dull right-sided lower abdominal pain and spotting of blood per vagina. The mother insists her daughter is a virgin. On examination temperature 36.5°C, BP 90/50 and pulse 120/min. The lower abdomen is rigid with rebound tenderness in the right iliac fossa. Her period is overdue. The MOST appropriate management following resuscitation is

A Ask to speak to the girl in private, and obtain confidential information from her as to whether she has been sexually-active. If so, perform a urinanalysis, urine β-HCG pregnancy test and pelvic exam with triple swabs.
B Arrange for urgent transvaginal ultrasound to exclude ectopic pregnancy.
C Accept that the daughter is a virgin, omit a pelvic internal exam and take a low vaginal swab to exclude infection.
D Arrange for pelvic ultrasound to exclude ectopic pregnancy and acute appendicitis.
E Inform the mother that you are performing a urine pregnancy test in the best interests of her daughter to exclude possibility of a miscarriage or ectopic pregnancy.

98. A 30-year-old woman presents with a spiking temperature and a foul-smelling vaginal discharge 24 hours after delivery of her baby. She has been sexually active with her partner throughout the pregnancy. The MOST likely organism is

A group A streptococcus
B group B streptococcus
C *Chlamydia trachomatis*
D *Gardnerella vaginalis*
E *Neisseria gonorrhoea*

99. *Neisseria gonorrhoea* may infect all of the following areas EXCEPT

A vagina
B rectum
C pharynx
D conjunctiva
E urethra

100. The following statements regarding *Chlamydia trachomatis* are correct EXCEPT

A It is the commonest cause of non-gonococcal urethritis.
B It is more often symptomatic in women.
C It causes Reiter's syndrome.
D It is treated with doxycycline.
E It causes perihepatitis.

Answers to Paper Three BOFs

Criterion Referencing Marks

* – 25–50% of candidates expected to get correct
** – 50–75% of candidates expected to get correct
*** – 75–100% of candidates expected to get correct

The notional PASS MARK is 71%

1. B **

2. E *** Chlamydia infection is treated with doxycycline.

3. A **

4. C *** The diagnosis of alcoholic hepatitis should be confirmed by liver biopsy.

5. B **

6. D ** Carcinomatous meningitis is associated with the presence of mononuclear cells.

7. C * Hand foot and mouth disease is caused by Coxsackie A16 virus.

8. B ***

9. B *** Fibroids are associated with menorrhagia.

10. B ***

11. C ***

12. A ** Amodarone is a class III anti-arrhythmic drug.

13. C ***

14. C *

15. B *** Lidocaine (lignocaine) is a second-line drug for treatment of refractory ventricular fibrillation.

16. C *** Digoxin decreases the conduction velocity in the Purkinje fibres.

17. C * Arrhythmias associated with TCA poisoning should respond to correction of hypoxia and acidosis.

18. A * Forced alkaline diuresis is no longer recommended by the British National Formulary (BNF).

19. B *** Donepezil is used to treat Alzheimer's disease.

20. A * Ethosuximide and sodium valproate are the drugs of choice in the treatment of absence seizures.

21. B *** This man has Wegener's granulomatosis.

22. A **

23. D *

24. D **

25. B ***

26. C ***

27. D ** Acute coronary syndrome also includes non-Q-wave MI, unstable angina and Q-wave MI.

28. A **

29. A ** The internal jugular vein initially lies behind the carotid artery in the neck.

30. A ** Adrenaline (epinephrine) is given by IV infusion and not by bolus. Pacing is performed on the R wave and not the T wave. The latter would kill the patient!

31. C ***

32. B ***

33. B ***

34. A *** ECG changes in cor pulmonale include P pulmonale, RAD, RVH and inverted T waves in V1—4. The chest x-ray and sputum may be normal. Lung function tests will show airflow obstruction. Arterial blood gases will confirm hypoxia and show degree of hypercapnia which is important in guiding management.

35. A ***

36. D **

37. E *** OSA is associated with carbon dioxide retention and may manifest as morning headaches.

38. A ***

39. B * Needle cricothyroidotomy may be necessary as an emergency procedure in casualty. The leading cause of death from glandular fever (infectious mononucleosis) is failed endotracheal intubation! Bear in mind that the patient has jaw trismus! Needle cricothyroidotomy will buy time for tracheostomy by an ENT surgeon in theatre.

40. A ***

41. C ***

42. A *** This is classic farmer's lung. Dairy farmers require hay to feed their cows.

43. B ** Pulmonary embolism is a cause of physiological dead space.

44. C **

45. E **

46. E *** Sulphur granules are associated with actinomycosis.

47. E ***

48. B **

49. C ***

50. A **

51. B *

52. D ***

53. B **

54. A **

55. D * This patient has acute angle closure glaucoma. Pupils dilate at dusk which close off the angle. Visual loss can result from use of dilators! IV Diamox (acetazolamide) is recommended to reduce pressures. This patient has 6–8 hours before impending visual loss and requires urgent referral.

56. B ***

57. E **

58. C ***

59. D ***

60. C ***

61. B ***

62. A *

63. B ***

64. A *** This man presents with signs of colorectal carcinoma. Colonoscopy is an alternative investigation.

65. B ***

66. E **

67. A *** The patient exhibits Charcot's triad.

68. B **

69. B **

70. E ***

71. E ** Bone metastases are usually associated with low albumin and increased alkaline phosphatase.

72. E ***

73. E ***

74. C ***

75. E ** Flail chest is associated with respiratory acidosis.

76. D ** Gram-negative sepsis is associated with mixed metabolic acidosis and respiratory alkalosis.

77. C **

78. D **

79. A **

80. A ** Hyperprolactinaemia may occur in hypothyroidism not hyperthyroidism.

81. C ** Primary hypoparathyroidism is associated with neck surgery.

82. B **

83. D ***

84. C ***

85. E ***

86. C ***

87. D * Hyperparathyroidism is associated with distal renal tubular acidosis.

88. C ***

89. B **

90. B ***

91. E * The organism is the yeast *Pityrosporum orbiculare*.

92. A **

93. E ***

94. A ***

95. E **

96. E **

97. A *

98. B **

99. A * *Neisseria gonorrhoea* affects columnar epithelium. The vagina is composed of squamous epithelium. This explains why the endocervix and not the vagina is swabbed for the presence of the organism.

100. B ** Chlamydia is often asymptomatic in women.

MRCP Paper Four BOFs

In these questions candidates must select one answer only

Questions

1. *Toxoplasma gondii* infection in patients with AIDS may present with any of the following EXCEPT

   A chorioretinitis
   B seizures
   C myocarditis
   D hepatitis
   E encephalitis

2. The organism responsible for gas gangrene IS

   A *Clostridium difficile*
   B *Clostridium perfringens*
   C *Clostridium tetanus*
   D *Klebsiella* sp.
   E *Pseudomonas aeruginosa*

3. The following diseases are associated with the Ebstein–Barr virus EXCEPT

   A craniopharyngioma
   B Burkitt's lymphoma
   C sinonasal tumours
   D glandular fever
   E Hodgkin's lymphoma

4. Shock is associated with all of the following changes EXCEPT

   A increased protein metabolism
   B decreased free fatty acids
   C increased liver glycogenolysis
   D increased uric acid
   E increased lactic production

5. A 60-year-old man presents with dementia. He has a past history of a subarachnoid haemorrhage. He is noted to suffer from urinary incontinence and apraxia. He walks with an unsteady gait. The MOST likely diagnosis is

A lacunar infarct
B normal pressure hydrocephalus
C Creutzfeldt–Jakob syndrome
D lateral medullary syndrome
E progressive multifocal leuco-encephalopathy

6. Typhoid fever is associated with all of the following EXCEPT

A bowel perforation
B splenomegaly
C ulceration of Peyer's patches
D non-blanching maculopapular rash
E osteomyelitis

7. A 20-year-old man who has travelled recently to India presents with unexplained fever for 5 days. You suspect typhoid fever. The MOST appropriate investigation would be

A Widal test measuring serum levels of agglutinins to O and H antigens
B blood culture
C marrow culture
D stool culture
E urine culture

8. Risk factors predisposing to infection with candidiasis include all of the following EXCEPT

A poor T-lymphocyte function
B hyperalimentation
C diabetes mellitus
D broad-spectrum antibiotic therapy
E multiple sex partners

9. The following organisms and disease are correctly paired EXCEPT

A *Streptococcus pyogenes* – necrotising fasciitis
B *Staphylococcus epidermidis* – toxic shock syndrome
C *Staphylococcus aureus* – scalded skin syndrome
D *Staphylococcus aureus* – impetigo
E *Streptococcus pyogenes* – acute rheumatic fever

10. Haemolytic anaemia is associated with all of the following EXCEPT

    A increased urinary urobilinogen
    B decreased haptoglobin
    C urinary haemosiderin
    D positive indirect Coombs' test
    E increased unconjugated bilirubin

11. A 25-year-old woman self-prescribes vitamins and iron tablets. She presents with acute abdominal pain. She is found to be pancytopenic with haemosiderin in her urine and trace haemoglobin. The MOST likely diagnosis is

    A SLE
    B aplastic anaemia
    C myelofibrosis
    D paroxysmal nocturnal haemoglobinuria
    E acute myeloid leukaemia

12. A 20-year-old pregnant black woman presents with fever and joint pains. She has a history of two previous spontaneous early miscarriages. Her urine reveals 2+ protein. Her blood results show leucopenia, normocytic normochromic anaemia and thrombocytopenia. The MOST likely diagnosis is

    A sickle cell disease
    B SLE
    C thalassaemia
    D aplastic anaemia
    E pre-eclampsia

13. A 60-year-old woman presents with morning stiffness in both knees and pain worse at the end of the day. On examination the knees are swollen and warm to the touch with a flexion deformity and limitation of movement. X-ray shows narrowing of the joint spaces, osteophytes at the margin of the joints and sclerosis of the underlying bone. Recognised treatment for this condition includes all of the following EXCEPT

    A total knee replacement
    B NSAIDs
    C penicillamine
    D intra-articular corticosteroid
    E physiotherapy

14. The MOST useful investigation for her miscarriages would be

A transvaginal ultrasound
B chromosome karyotype
C lupus anticoagulant and anticardiolipin antibody
D hysterosalpingogram
E antithrombin III, protein C and S deficiency

15. The following statements regarding haemoglobin are correct EXCEPT

A It consists of 2 globin subunits containing a single haem molecule.
B Haem consists of a porphyrin ring and one atom of iron.
C δ-aminolaevulinic acid (ALA) synthetase is the rate-controlling enzyme in haem synthesis.
D Haem is catabolised to biliverdin.
E Conjugated bilirubin is hydrolysed and the free pigment is reduced to urobilinogen and stercobilinogen in the gut.

16. The following statements regarding transplantation are correct EXCEPT

A The cornea is the most commonly transplanted allograft.
B Nephrectomy is required prior to kidney transplantation in Goodpasture's syndrome.
C Recent malignancy in the recipient is a contraindication to transplantation.
D The most common cause of death in patients with transplants is malignancy.
E Reticulum cell sarcoma is common in recipients.

17. A 35-year-old African woman is found to have a Hb of 6g/dL. She is a vegetarian and has a history of uterine fibroids. Her blood film reveals microcytic, hypochromic red blood cells and a few target cells. The MOST likely result of iron studies would be

A low ferritin, high TIBC
B low iron, low TIBC
C raised ferritin, low TIBC
D low serum iron, low TIBC
E normal ferritin, high TIBC

18. The following statements regarding immunosuppressive therapy are correct EXCEPT

A Tacrolimus is a calcineurin agonist.
B Rituximab is used in treatment of chemotherapy-resistant advanced follicular lymphoma.
C Ciclosporin is associated with hypertension in heart transplant patients.
D Gingival hyperplasia is a recognised side-effect of ciclosporin.
E Basiliximab is used for prophylaxis of acute rejection in allogenic renal transplantation.

19. Delayed alloimmunisation by previous blood transfusions is associated with all of the following EXCEPT

A destruction of transfused blood cells by IgM antibodies
B spherocytosis
C reticulocytosis
D positive direct antiglobulin test
E extravascular haemolysis

20. The following statements regarding terfenadine are correct EXCEPT

A Patients are advised to avoid grapefruit juice.
B Ventricular arrhythmias have followed excessive dosage.
C It has been associated with erythema multiforme.
D It should be used cautiously in patients with liver disease.
E It causes marked sedation because it penetrates the blood brain barrier.

21. The following statements regarding octreotide are correct EXCEPT

A It is a somatostatin antagonist.
B It may cause gallstones.
C It may be valuable in cessation of variceal bleeding.
D Abrupt withdrawal is associated with pancreatitis.
E It is indicated for the relief of symptoms associated with carcinoid tumours.

22. A 50-year-old farmer presents with acute shortness of breath, dizziness and severe headache. His skin is red in colour, and he smells of bitter almonds. He mentions that he had been using rodenticides. His condition rapidly deteriorates. The MOST appropriate treatment for him would be

A atropine
B sodium nitrite and sodium thiosulphate
C vitamin K
D dimercaprol
E activated charcoal

23. The following statements regarding tetracyclines are correct EXCEPT

A They are broad-spectrum bacteriocidal antibiotics.
B Demeclocycline may cause reversible nephrogenic diabetes insipidus.
C Absorption is decreased by milk and antacids except for doxycycline.
D They cause dental discolouration and hypoplasia in children.
E They are the drug of choice for non-gonococcal urethritis.

24. The following statements regarding paracetamol poisoning are correct EXCEPT

A Acetylcysteine protects the liver if given 24 hours after ingestion.
B Activated charcoal is administered if ingestion of 150 mg/kg occurred within the hour.
C It may cause renal tubular necrosis.
D Maximum liver damage occurs 3–4 days following ingestion.
E Patients on enzyme-inducing drugs may develop toxicity at lower plasma-paracetamol concentrations.

25. Hepatic microsomal enzyme-inducing drugs include all of the following EXCEPT

A phenytoin
B carbamazepine
C rifampicin
D alcohol
E warfarin

26. The following statements regarding aminoglycosides are correct EXCEPT

A They are bactericidal antibiotics.
B They are well absorbed from the gut.
C Side-effects include ototoxicity and nephrotoxicity.
D Neomycin is used to reduce colonic bacterial flora in patients with hepatic failure.
E They cross the placenta and may cause fetal VIIIth nerve damage.

27. The following statements regarding antiviral drugs are correct EXCEPT

A Valaciclovir is indicated for treatment of recurrent genital herpes.
B Peripheral neuropathy is a side-effect of didanosine.
C Zidovudine is indicated as monotherapy for prevention of maternal-fetal HIV transmission.
D Parkinsonism is a side-effect of amantadine.
E Ganciclovir is active against cytomegalovirus.

28. The following statements regarding antithyroid drugs are correct EXCEPT

A Carbimazole may induce bone marrow suppression.
B Radioactive sodium iodide is safe in patients with heart disease.
C Propylthiouracil (PTU) does not cross the placenta.
D Carbimazole may be associated with alopecia.
E PTU is associated with aplastic anaemia.

29. A 20-year-old man complains of recurrent lower back pain and stiffness after exercise. He has no morning stiffness. His full blood count and ESR are normal, but he is found to have HLA-B27. X-ray of his lumbar spine and pelvis are normal. The MOST appropriate management would be

A no further investigations and reassure the patient that HLA-B27 can also be found in normal people
B arrange for an ophthalmology referral for slit-lamp examination
C arrange a Kveim test to exclude sarcoidosis
D arrange for barium follow-through
E test for rheumatoid factor

30. Major criteria for the diagnosis of rheumatic fever include all of the following EXCEPT

A polyarthralgia
B chorea
C erythema marginatum
D subcutaneous nodules
E fever

31. The following HLA antigens and diseases have been correctly paired EXCEPT

A HLA-B27 – Reiter's syndrome
B HLA-B14 and A3 – multiple sclerosis
C HLA-DR4 – rheumatoid arthritis
D HLA-DR3 – idiopathic membranous glomerulonephritis
E HLA-DR2 – Goodpasture's syndrome

32. The following statements regarding juvenile rheumatoid arthritis are correct EXCEPT

A It has a worse prognosis than in adults.
B It is usually associated with a positive rheumatoid factor.
C It may occur before the 16th birthday.
D Clinical features are the same as those in adults.
E It is the most common type of juvenile chronic arthritis.

33. The following statements regarding urate metabolism are correct EXCEPT

A Thiazide diuretics impair urate secretion in the renal tubules.
B Leukaemia and polycythaemia both increase nucleic acid turnover.
C Allopurinol increases the activity of xanthine oxidase.
D Probenecid acts by inhibition of tubular reabsorption of urate.
E Glucose-6-phosphatase deficiency results in increased urate production.

34. A 38-year-old man presents with painful right wrist and left knee joint a fortnight after an attack of gastroenteritis. Prostatic massage produces a urethral discharge. The synovial fluid shows an abundance of neutrophils and is sterile. The ESR is raised. The MOST likely diagnosis is

A gonococcal arthritis
B rheumatoid arthritis
C salmonella arthritis
D Reiter's syndrome
E viral arthritis

35. The MOST appropriate treatment for this man would be

A amoxicillin
B non-steroidal anti-inflammatory drug
C penicillin
D gold
E doxycycline

36. The following statements regarding sarcoidosis are correct EXCEPT

A There is a higher incidence among young black males than caucasians.
B It most commonly involves the mediastinal lymph nodes.
C A third of cases are associated with erythema nodosum.
D Scalene node biopsy will be positive in 90% of cases.
E A negative Kveim test excludes sarcoidosis.

37. The MOST common organism implicated in infective endocarditis is

A Staphylococcus aureus
B Streptococcus viridans
C Streptococcus faecalis
D Staphylococcus epidermidis
E Coxiella burnetii

38. A 25-year-old heroin addict presents with fever and mucosal petechial haemorrhages. On examination he has a pansystolic murmur best heard at the lower sternal edge. He is also noted to have small, flat, erythematous, non-tender macules over the thenar eminence. The MOST likely diagnosis is

A subacute bacterial endocarditis
B acute bacterial endocarditis
C rheumatic heart disease
D acute rheumatic fever
E Q fever

39. The following statements regarding verapamil are correct EXCEPT

A It belongs to the class IV anti-arrhythmic drugs.
B It reduces the plateau phase of the action potential.
C It is indicated for supraventricular tachycardia.
D It is contraindicated in the presence of β-blockers.
E It may precipitate digoxin toxicity.

40. The following pulse patterns are correctly matched with their disorders EXCEPT

A pulsus alternans – left ventricular failure
B pulsus paradoxus – cardiac tamponade
C pulsus bisferiens – hypertrophic obstructive cardiomyopathy
D pulsus parvus et tardus (small volume, slow rising) – aortic regurgitation
E dicrotic pulse – dilated cardiomyopathy

41. A 70-year-old man presents with dyspnoea and chest pain. His pulse rate is 120, and he is extremely agitated. His arterial blood gas reveals low arterial oxygen and low CO_2. His ECG shows S wave in I, Q wave in III and T wave inversion in leads V1–3. The MOST likely diagnosis is

A myocardial infarction
B pulmonary embolism
C acute pericarditis
D cardiac tamponade
E pneumothorax

42. A 25-year-old healthy male smoker presents with gangrene of the left big toe. There are no signs of external trauma. The MOST likely diagnosis is

A thromboangiitis obliterans (Buerger's disease)
B Raynaud's disease
C gas gangrene
D polyarteritis nodosa
E gout

43. Bilharzia is associated with all of the following EXCEPT

A portal hypertension
B Asian Katayama fever
C haematuria
D type III hypersensitivity reaction
E tropical pulmonary eosinophilia

44. The following statements regarding leukotriene receptor antagonists are correct EXCEPT

A Churg–Strauss syndrome has been associated with use of these antagonists following the reduction or withdrawal of oral corticosteroid therapy.
B Zafirlukast is indicated for the prophylaxis of asthma.
C Montelukast may be used as add-on therapy in severe asthma.
D They block the effect of cysteinyl leukotrienes in the airways.
E Montelukast may be used to prevent exercise-induced bronchospasm.

45. Cystic fibrosis is associated with all of the following EXCEPT

A abnormal gene coding for transmembrane regulating factor protein on chromosome 7
B allergic bronchopulmonary aspergillosis
C steatorrhoea
D chronic infection with *Pseudomonas pseudomallei*
E diabetes mellitus

46. The following statements regarding lung function tests are correct EXCEPT

A Total lung capacity = vital capacity + residual volume.
B A normal transfer factor in the presence of persistently reduced FEV_1 may occur with chronic asthma.
C In restrictive lung diseases the FEV_1 to FVC ratio is higher than normal.
D Transfer factor measures gas transfer by assessing carbon monoxide uptake.
E Peak flows in flow volume loops are most affected at high volumes in distal obstruction.

47. Contraindications to surgery for lung carcinoma include all of the following EXCEPT

   A phrenic nerve involvement
   B superior vena cava obstruction
   C oat cell carcinoma
   D FEV_1 1.8 L
   E recurrent laryngeal nerve palsy

48. A 60-year-old dairy farmer presents with fever, cough and shortness of breath. Coarse end-inspiratory crackles are present. Chest x-ray shows bilateral fluffy nodular shadows. The MOST appropriate treatment is

   A amphotericin
   B prednisolone
   C cyclophosphamide
   D salbutamol
   E ciprofloxacin

49. A 40-year-old long-stay patient in a psychiatric hospital presents with fever, abdominal pain, dry cough and worsening confusion. Blood tests reveal neutrophilia, lymphopaenia and hyponatraemia. Chest x-ray shows right-sided lobar consolidation. The MOST appropriate treatment would be

   A erythromycin
   B benzylpenicillin
   C antituberculous chemotherapy
   D ciprofloxacin
   E ticarcillin

50. A 70-year-old man presents with chronic cough, haemoptysis and weight loss. He smokes 20 cigarettes a day. His chest x-ray shows a central coin lesion. The MOST useful investigation would be

   A sputum for culture and cytology
   B isotope bone scan
   C bronchoscopy and biopsy
   D percutaneous needle biopsy
   E chest CT scan

51. A 70-year-old man presents with progressive stepwise dementia associated with focal neurological events. He has a stiff, slow-moving, spastic tongue, dysarthria and inappropriate laughing and crying. He walks with a shuffling gait taking small steps. He is also noted to be hypertensive. The MOST likely diagnosis is

A Parkinson's disease
B Alzheimer's disease
C multi-infarct dementia
D variant CJD (BSE related)
E multiple sclerosis

52. The following are types of viral haemorrhagic fever EXCEPT

A yellow fever
B Lassa fever
C Dengue fever
D Ebola virus
E relapsing fever

53. Injury to the upper trunk of the brachial plexus affects the following muscles EXCEPT

A deltoid
B serratus anterior
C brachioradialis
D triceps
E infraspinatus

54. Charcot's joints are a recognised feature of all the following conditions EXCEPT

A leprosy
B diabetes mellitus
C syringomyelia
D syphilis
E rheumatoid arthritis

55. Which ONE of the following features would favour a diagnosis of Guillain–Barré syndrome rather than myasthenia gravis

A ocular muscle involvement
B proximal muscle weakness
C respiratory difficulties
D areflexia
E facial muscle weakness

56. Treatment for multiple sclerosis and its complications includes all of the following EXCEPT

A glatiramer acetate
B botulinum toxin
C interferon beta
D interferon alfa
E baclofen

57. The following neurovascular structures and injuries are correctly paired EXCEPT

A tibial nerve – proximal fibula fracture
B sciatic nerve – posterior dislocation of the hip
C median nerve – Smith's wrist fracture
D axillary nerve – fracture to humeral neck
E brachial artery – supracondylar fracture of the humerus

58. Radial nerve injury is associated with all of the following EXCEPT

A wrist drop
B weakness of the brachioradialis muscle
C loss of supinator reflex
D inability to abduct thumb to 90° to palm
E wasting of abductor pollicis brevis

59. A 20-year-old man presents with pain on eye movement and double vision after being punched in the eye. On examination he has limitation of upward gaze and anaesthesia over the lateral face and nose. The following injuries are possible EXCEPT

A blowout fracture
B inferior rectus entrapment
C infraorbital nerve injury
D retinal detachment
E increased intraorbital pressure

60. The cause of gradual bilateral loss of vision is LEAST likely to be

A cataract
B optic atrophy
C diabetic retinopathy
D chronic glaucoma
E choroiditis

61. Eye signs associated with Grave's disease include all of the following EXCEPT

A exophthalmos
B proptosis
C external ophthalmoplegia
D supraorbital and infraorbital swelling
E ptosis

62. Recognised treatment for mania include all of the following EXCEPT

A phenelzine
B chlorpromazine
C carbamazepine
D haloperidol
E lithium

63. The following are symptoms of schizophrenia EXCEPT

A obsessional intrusive thoughts
B thought insertion
C poverty of speech
D suspiciousness
E primary delusion

64. Psychiatric symptoms occur in all of the following physical diseases EXCEPT

A puerperal infection
B leprosy
C nicotinic acid deficiency
D pernicious anaemia
E normal pressure hydrocephalus

65. A 20-year-old woman presents with arthralgia and acute jaundice. Markers for hepatitis B infection at this stage could include all of the following EXCEPT

A HBeAg
B HBsAg
C IgM anti-HBc
D Anti-HBe
E Anti-HBs

66. Coeliac disease is associated with all of the following EXCEPT

   A vitamin B_{12} deficiency
   B HLA DR3
   C dermatitis herpetiformis
   D steatorrhoea
   E lymphoma

67. Crohn's disease is commonly associated with all of the following EXCEPT

   A gallstones
   B acute ileitis
   C sclerosing cholangitis
   D aphthous ulceration
   E hyperoxaluria

68. The following statements regarding the management of hepatocellular carcinoma (HCC) are correct EXCEPT

   A Partial hepatectomy is the mainstay therapy for early HCC.
   B Hepatitis B infection is a contraindication to liver transplantation.
   C Percutaneous ethanol injection is the most commonly used form of local ablative therapy.
   D Transarterial embolisation is relatively contraindicated if the portal system is blocked by tumour invasion.
   E HCC is relatively resistant to systemic chemotherapy.

69. Which ONE of the following features would favour a diagnosis of ulcerative colitis rather than Crohn's disease?

   A uveitis
   B arthritis
   C pyoderma gangrenosum
   D cholelithiasis
   E pseudopolyps

70. Peptic ulcer disease is associated with all of the following EXCEPT

   A head trauma
   B burns
   C chronic pancreatitis
   D hypocalcaemia
   E helicobacter antral gastritis

71. The following statements regarding bile acids are correct EXCEPT

A They are absorbed in the ileum.
B They combine with glycine and taurine to form bile salts.
C In the intestine they emulsify fats.
D Cholic acid is a secondary bile acid.
E Cholesterol is a precursor of the bile acids.

72. The following are causes of megacolon EXCEPT

A poliomyelitis
B Whipple's disease
C Chagas' disease
D laxative abuse
E systemic sclerosis

73. The following statements regarding juvenile colonic polyps are correct EXCEPT

A They are pre-malignant.
B Most disappear prior to adulthood.
C They are rarely symptomatic.
D They are usually in the sigmoid colon.
E They may be complicated by rectal prolapse.

74. A 50-year-old woman presents with watery diarrhoea and right iliac fossa pain. On examination a rumbling mid-diastolic murmur is auscultated at the lower left sternal border, louder on inspiration, and the liver is enlarged. 12-lead ECG shows peaked, tall P waves in lead II. The MOST likely diagnosis is

A VIPoma
B phaeochromocytoma
C gastrinoma
D carcinoid syndrome
E MEN type I syndrome

75. Sites of carcinoid tumours include all of the following EXCEPT

A appendix
B terminal ileum
C bronchus
D oesophagus
E rectum

76. The MOST common cause of significant upper gastrointestinal bleeding is

   A gastric ulcer
   B duodenal ulcer
   C oesophageal varices
   D Mallory–Weiss syndrome
   E angiodysplasia

77. Recognised causes of massive splenomegaly include all of the following EXCEPT

   A malaria
   B bilharzia
   C idiopathic thrombocytopaenic purpura
   D myelofibrosis
   E chronic myeloid leukaemia

78. Risk factors associated with hepatocellular carcinoma include all of the following EXCEPT

   A smoking
   B *Clonorchis sinensis*
   C vinyl chloride
   D aflatoxins
   E hepatitis B

79. The following statements regarding vitamin D are correct EXCEPT

   A 1,25 (OH)$_2$ D3 is the most active form.
   B 25 (OH) D3 stimulates both calcium and phosphorus absorption in the intestine and the resorption of calcium from bone.
   C Cholecalciferol is synthesised in the skin through the actions of sunlight on 7-dehydrochloesterol.
   D The production of 1,25 (OH)$_2$ D3 is regulated by parathyroid hormone.
   E The measurement of 25(OH) D3 is a good indicator of vitamin D bioavailability.

80. A 55-year-old insulin-dependent diabetic presents with nausea, lethargy, dry and itchy yellow-brown skin. He also complains of nocturia and impotence. Blood film shows normocytic normochromic anaemia and occasional burr cells. The MOST appropriate management would be

   A Commence iron replacement therapy.
   B Take blood for urea and electrolytes.
   C Check HbA1C.
   D Take blood for bilirubin, LFTs and amylase.
   E Take blood for thyroid function tests.

81. A 20-year-old female presents with acne and hirsutism. She complains of a year of chaotic menstrual cycles with long periods of amenorrhoea. She has gained weight recently. She has never been pregnant. On examination there are no other abnormalities. The MOST likely diagnosis is

A congenital adrenal hyperplasia
B ovarian teratoma
C Cushing's disease
D testicular feminisation
E polycystic ovarian syndrome

82. The type of thyroid carcinoma with the HIGHEST 10-year survival rate is

A follicular
B anaplastic
C medullary
D squamous
E papillary

83. A 50-year-old man presents with polydipsia, headache and weakness. On examination BP is 160/100 but he is not oedematous. He takes no medication. Blood results reveal hypokalaemia, alkalosis and low serum renin. The MOST likely diagnosis is

A Conn's syndrome
B secondary hyperaldosteronism
C Cushing's disease
D phaeochromocytoma
E renal artery stenosis

84. The following statements regarding gastrin are correct EXCEPT

A It stimulates parietal cells to secrete HCL acid.
B Secretin inhibits gastrin release.
C Somatostatin enhances the release of gastrin.
D It is secreted by G cells in the antrum.
E Duodenal distension enhances the release of gastrin.

85. Functions of cholecystokinin include all of the following EXCEPT

A gallbladder contraction
B pancreatic enzyme secretion
C contraction of the sphincter of Oddi
D inhibition of gastric emptying
E jejunal mucosal enzyme secretion (succus entericus)

86. A patient presents with polydipsia and polyuria, up to 10 L/day. First morning urine osmolality is 300 mosm/kg. Plasma osmolality is high. He undergoes a water deprivation test. The plasma osmolality rises but the urine osmolality remains dilute. Following desmopressin, the urine osmolality rises to 450 mosm/kg. The MOST likely diagnosis is

A nephrogenic diabetes insipidus
B psychogenic diabetes insipidus
C cranial diabetes insipidus
D SIADH
E diabetes mellitus

87. The following statements regarding vasopressin are correct EXCEPT

A It is synthesised in the posterior pituitary gland.
B It increases peristalsis.
C It increases resorption of water from the distal renal tubules.
D It causes coronary artery vasoconstriction.
E It causes reduction in portal pressure.

88. Precocious puberty may be associated with all of the following EXCEPT

A hepatoma
B adrenal tumour
C McCune–Albright's syndrome
D Klinefelter's syndrome
E ovarian tumour

89. The following results

increased serum calcium
increased serum phosphate
decreased parathyroid hormone (PTH)
increased urinary calcium
increased urinary phosphate

are compatible with which ONE diagnosis?

A vitamin D toxicity
B carcinomatosis
C primary hyperparathyroidism
D secondary hyperparathyroidism
E milk alkali syndrome

90. Diseases associated with impotence include all of the following EXCEPT

A hyperthyroidism
B hyperprolactinaemia
C cirrhosis
D multiple sclerosis
E renal failure

91. The following statements regarding thyroid hormones are correct EXCEPT

A In blood, thyroxine and triiodothyronine are almost entirely bound to plasma proteins.
B Thyroid stimulating hormone (TSH) stimulates the TSH receptor in the thyroid to release stored hormone.
C 0.03% of T4 is free hormone.
D The metabolic state correlates with the total amount of hormone in plasma.
E 30% of T4 is converted to T3.

92. A 30-year-old dark-tanned man presents with progressive weakness, anorexia, diarrhoea and weight loss. He has just returned from holiday in Cyprus. On examination: BP 100/60. He is noted to have mucosal bluish-black plaques. Blood results:

serum sodium	130 mmol/L
serum potassium	5 mmol/L
serum calcium	3 mmol/L
serum creatinine	200 µmol/L
serum urea	8 mmol/L

The MOST likely diagnosis is

A Addison's disease
B primary hyperparathyroidism
C SIADH
D thyrotoxicosis
E heavy metal poisoning

93. Characteristic features of distal renal tubular acidosis include all of the following EXCEPT

A hypokalaemia
B inability to acidify the urine below pH 5.5
C hypercalciuria
D nephrolithiasis
E association with Fanconi syndrome

94. The MOST common cause of painless frank haematuria in male patients over 50 years old is

A bladder squamous cell carcinoma
B carcinoma of the prostate
C hypernephroma
D transitional cell carcinoma in the kidney
E transitional cell bladder carcinoma

95. A 30-year-old man presents to Casualty with a tender swollen testicle. He states that he was struck in the groin while playing football. On examination the border of the testicle is irregular, and the testicle is heavy and woody. There is no associated lymphadenopathy. He is also noted to have gynaecomastia. There are no external signs of trauma. The MOST appropriate initial management would be

A take blood for α fetoprotein and β-HCG and arrange for a chest x-ray
B prescribe doxycycline 100 mg o bd × 5 days
C refer to urologists for urgent surgical exploration
D arrange for a chest and abdominal CT scan
E arrange for an ultrasound of the testes

96. The following statements regarding renal tubular disease are correct EXCEPT

A Hypophosphataemic rickets is due to distal renal tubular unresponsiveness to vitamin D.
B Cystinosis is associated with proximal renal tubular acidosis (RTA).
C Osteomalacia is associated with distal RTA.
D Type I or distal RTA occurs when the tubules fail to create an acid urine.
E Renal transplantation is associated with proximal RTA.

97. Alport's syndrome is associated with all of the following EXCEPT

A autosomal dominant inheritance
B high-frequency sensorineural hearing loss
C cataract formation
D bone pain
E renal tubular disease

98. Cutaneous manifestations of internal malignancy include all the following EXCEPT

A acquired ichthyosis
B dermatomyositis
C thrombophlebitis migrans
D mycosis fungoides
E vitiligo

99. Systemic effects of a major burn include all of the following EXCEPT

A decrease in pulmonary vascular resistance
B decrease in cardiac output in early burn
C red cell destruction
D duodenal mucosa ulceration
E extravascular fluid and protein loss

100. Type I (von Recklinghausen's) neurofibromatosis is associated with all of the following EXCEPT

A autosomal dominant inheritance
B café-au-lait spots
C acoustic neuromas
D honeycomb lung
E axillary freckling

Answers to Paper Four BOFs

Criterion Referencing Marks

*   – 25–50% of candidates expected to get correct
* *   – 50–75% of candidates expected to get correct
* * * – 75–100% of candidates expected to get correct

The notional PASS MARK is 69%

1. A ** The tetrad of Sabin is associated with congenital toxoplasmosis (internal hydrocephalus or microcephaly, chorioretinitis, convulsions and cerebral calcification).

2. B ***

3. C **

4. B ** Shock is associated with increased FFAs.

5. B **

6. D *** Rose spots blanch under pressure.

7. B **

8. E **

9. B ** *Staphylococcus aureus* is the organism responsible for toxic shock syndrome.

10. D ** Haemolytic anaemia is associated with a positive direct Coombs' test.

11. D *

12. B ***

13. C *** Penicillamine is a form of treatment for rheumatoid arthritis.

14. C ***

15. A ** Haemoglobin consists of 4 globin subunits containing a single haem molecule.

16. D ** The most common cause of death in transplants is from infection.

17. A **

18. A * Tacrolimus is a calcineurin inhibitor.

19. A ** It is associated with destruction of transfused blood cells by IgG antibodies.

20. E *

21. A ** Octreotide is a somatostatin analogue.

22. B **

23. A ** Tetracycline is a bacteriostatic antibiotic.

24. A ***

25. E **

26. B ***

27. D ** Amantadine is also used to treat Parkinsonism.

28. C **

29. B **

30. E **

31. B ** HLA-B14 and HLA-A3 are associated with idiopathic haemochromatosis.

32. E ** Still's disease is the most common form of juvenile chronic arthritis.

33. C ** Allopurinol is a competitive xanthine oxidase inhibitor.

34. D ***

35. B ***

36. E ***

37. B ***

38. B *** The palmar macules described are Janeway lesions.

39. D ** Verapamil may be used in the presence of β-blockers but with caution to avoid refractory hypotension.

40. D ** Pulsus parvus et tardus is associated with aortic stenosis.

41. B ***

42. A ***

43. D ** Bilharzia is associated with a Type IV hypersensitivity reaction.

44. C * Montelukast may be used in mild to moderate asthma.

45. D ** Cystic fibrosis is associated with chronic infection with *Pseudomonas aeruginosa*.

46. E ** Peak flows in flow volume loops are most affected at low volumes in distal obstruction such as asthma.

47. D ***

48. B ***

49. A ** Erythromycin is the recommended antibiotic for legionella.

50. C ***

51. C **

52. E **

53. D **

54. E ***

55. D **

56. D ** Glatiramer is a recently introduced immunomodulator.

57. A ** The common peroneal nerve is at risk with a fracture to the proximal neck of the fibula and manifests as a foot drop.

58. E ** Wasting of the abductor pollicis brevis is a sign of median nerve injury.

59. D *

60. E ** Choroiditis is associated with unilateral loss of vision.

61. E ***

62. A ***

63. A ***

64. B ***

65. E **

66. A ** Coeliac disease is associated with folate and iron deficiencies; even though some malabsorption of B_{12} may occur in the rarely involved terminal ileum it does not lead to deficiency of it.

67. C **

68. B * Hepatitis B is no longer a contraindication to liver transplantation with the advent of antiviral drugs such as lamivudine.

69. E ***

70. D *** Peptic ulcer disease is associated with hypercalcaemia not hypocalcaemia.

71. D ** Bile acids are synthesised and secreted by the liver into bile and converted to secondary bile acids in the small intestine (deoxycholic and lithocolic).

72. B **

73. A ** Juvenile colonic polyps have no malignant potential.

74. D ***

75. D **

76. B ***

77. C ***

78. A ***

79. B ** 1,25 (OH)$_2$ D3 stimulates both calicum and phosphorus absorption in the intestine and the resorption of calcium from bone.

80. B *** This patient has uraemia.

81. E ***

82. E ***

83. A ***

84. C **

85. C ** CCK relaxes the sphincter of Oddi.

86. C **

87. A ** Vasopressin is made in the hypothalamus and secreted by the posterior pituitary gland.

88. D **

89. A **

90. A ** Hypothyroidism and not hyperthyroidism is associated with impotence.

91. D **

92. A ***

93. E ** Fanconi syndrome is associated with proximal RTA.

94. E **

95. A **

96. A * Hypophosphataemic rickets is due to proximal tubular unresponsiveness to vitamin D.

97. D **

98. E **

99. A ** Major burns are associated with increased pulmonary vascular resistance and Curling's peptic ulcer.

100. C **

51/100

MRCP Paper Five BOFs

In these questions candidates must select one answer only

Questions

1. The following are transmitted by insect vectors EXCEPT

   A *Wucheria bancrofti*
   B *Plasmodium falciparum*
   C leishmania
   D *Trypanosoma brucei gambiense*
   E ascariasis

2. Pelvic inflammatory disease is associated with all of the following EXCEPT

   A infertility
   B ectopic pregnancies
   C *Chlamydia trachomatis* infection
   D tubo-ovarian abscess
   E endometriosis

3. The MOST common viral illness in transplant patients is

   A human immunodeficiency virus
   B herpes zoster
   C herpes simplex
   D cytomegalovirus
   E Epstein–Barr virus

4. A 20-year-old man returned from hitchhiking through South America a fortnight ago now presents with explosive watery foul-smelling diarrhoea and weight loss. On examination he has abdominal distension. His stools are greasy and contain mucus. The MOST useful investigation would be

   A proctoscopy
   B sodium sweat test
   C abdominal x-ray
   D stool for microscopy
   E duodenal aspirate

5. A 25-year-old man presents with a short history of fatigue and myalgia. The differential diagnosis includes all of the following EXCEPT

A cytomegalovirus
B infectious mononucleosis
C chronic fatigue syndrome (ME syndrome)
D toxoplasmosis
E prodromal herpes zoster

6. A 24-year-old African man presents to Casualty with acute onset of fever, vomiting, jaundice and dark brown-black urine. He had been travelling through Africa 6 weeks ago and had taken chloroquine prophylaxis. He is not taking any medication now. On examination he has irregular fever patterns and a BP 100/60. There is hepatosplenomegaly, hypertonia and hyper-reflexia. Serum urea and creatinine are markedly elevated and haemoglobinuria is present. The MOST likely diagnosis is

A *Plasmodium malariae*
B *Plasmodium falciparum*
C African trypanosomiasis
D yellow fever
E leishmaniasis

7. A 30-year-old man presents with fever and jaundice. He enjoys travelling and water sports and has recently returned from Sri Lanka. On examination he is also noted to have injected conjunctivae and hepatomegaly. His Hb is low, and he has microscopic haematuria. ESR, serum creatinine and urea are markedly raised, and his serum transaminases are only slightly raised. The MOST likely diagnosis is

A relapsing fever
B leptospira ictero haemorrhagica (Weil's disease)
C yellow fever
D Q fever
E leishmaniasis

8. A 30-year-old woman with Crohn's disease presents with left flank pain and microscopic haematuria. She admits she doesn't drink enough water. She smokes, drinks wine and loves chocolates. X-ray shows a radiopaque left renal calculus. Dietary recommendations you would make for her include avoidance of all of the following EXCEPT

A spinach
B rhubarb
C chocolate
D tomatoes
E tea

9. The following statements regarding Christmas disease are correct EXCEPT

A It is the second most common congenital coagulopathy.
B It is associated with Factor IX deficiency.
C It may be corrected with cryoprecipitate.
D It may cause severe bleeding post-injury.
E It may be corrected with fresh frozen plasma.

10. Primary tumours commonly associated with bone metastases include all of the following EXCEPT

A lymphoma
B breast
C prostate
D thyroid
E lung

11. Recognised complications of blood replacement by blood transfusion include all of the following EXCEPT

A hypothermia
B hyperkalaemia
C hypercalcaemia
D metabolic acidosis
E thrombocytopenia

12. Of the factors in Hodgkin's disease the one which carries the BEST prognosis is

A age greater than 50
B absence of constitutional symptoms
C lymphocyte depletion histologically
D female
E nodular sclerosis histologically

13. Chemical mediators of increased vascular permeability include all of the following EXCEPT

A C3b
B bradykinin
C histamine
D serotonin
E leukotriene

14. Post-splenectomy complications include all of the following EXCEPT

   A falciparum malaria
   B *Haemophilus influenzae* infection
   C pneumococcal septicaemia
   D thrombo-embolism
   E thrombocytopenia

15. The following antibiotics and mechanisms of action have been correctly paired EXCEPT

   A penicillin   inhibits cell wall synthesis
   B clavulanic acid   inhibits β-lactamase
   C erythromycin   inhibits protein synthesis in ribosome
   D gentamicin   inhibits folic acid synthesis
   E trimethoprim   inhibits dihydrofolate reductase

16. The following statements regarding ACE inhibitors are correct EXCEPT

   A ACE inhibitors are recommended within 24 hours of a myocardial infarction in a normotensive patient without any contraindications.
   B They should be avoided in insulin-dependent diabetics with nephropathy.
   C They are indicated for hypertension when thiazides and beta-blockers are contraindicated or have been less effective.
   D They should be used cautiously in patients receiving diuretics.
   E They cause severe renal failure in patients with bilateral renal artery stenosis.

17. The following statements regarding beta-blockers are correct EXCEPT

   A Carvedilol is recommended for patients with stable heart failure and left-ventricular systolic dysfunction.
   B Atenolol is contraindicated in NIDDM type II diabetes.
   C Sotalol is indicated for prophylaxis of paroxysmal atrial tachycardia.
   D Propranolol is contraindicated in patients with COPD.
   E Sudden withdrawal of propranolol may cause an exacerbation of angina.

18. The following antibiotics and their recognised complications have been correctly paired EXCEPT

   A chloramphenicol – aplastic anaemia
   B neomycin – nephrotoxicity
   C cephalosporin – bleeding dyscrasia
   D penicillin – bone marrow suppression
   E trimethoprim – teeth mottling

19. A 30-year-old man presents in coma following drug overdose. His pupils are dilated, and he is hypotensive. Pulse rate drops to 40 and ECG confirms second degree Mobitz type II heart block. The MOST likely cause of his overdose is

    A barbiturate
    B tricyclic antidepressant
    C lithium
    D beta-blocker
    E benzodiazepine

20. Recognised side-effects of thiazide diuretics include all of the following EXCEPT:

    A hyperuricaemia
    B increased LDL cholesterol
    C hypokalaemia
    D hypoglycaemia
    E hypercalcaemia

21. The first-line therapy for hypertension in a pregnant woman is

    A atenolol
    B hydralazine
    C methyldopa
    D bendrofluazide
    E nifedipine

22. The following are recognised treatment for migraine EXCEPT

    A methysergide
    B calcium-channel blocker
    C tricyclic antidepressant
    D beta-blocker
    E serotonin antagonist

23. The treatment of choice for adolescent-onset Gilles de la Tourette's syndrome is

    A ritalin
    B pimozide
    C haloperidol
    D clonidine
    E clonazepam

24. Sodium valproate is associated with all of the following EXCEPT

   A transient alopecia
   B Stevens–Johnson syndrome
   C ataxia
   D gynaecomastia
   E thrombocytosis

25. An 8-year-old recently adopted boy presents with painful swelling of the right knee. On examination there is joint subluxation and an effusion present. There is also wasting of the right quadriceps. Aspiration confirms haemarthrosis. The MOST likely diagnosis is

   A apophysitis of the tibial tubercle (Osgood–Schlatter disease)
   B haemophilia
   C juvenile rheumatoid arthritis
   D non-accidental injury (NAI)
   E Still's disease

26. A 40-year-old woman presents with fever, symmetrical polyar-thralgia affecting the fingers, wrists and knees, and weight loss. She is also noted to have alopecia, oral and nasal mucosal ulceration. Full blood count shows anaemia with thrombocytopenia. ESR is raised. The MOST definitive investigation is

   A rheumatoid factor
   B ANA
   C anticentromere antibodies
   D antibodies to double-stranded DNA
   E c-ANCA

27. A 15-year-old boy presents with high swinging fever and arthritis affecting the knees. The joints are swollen but not very tender. Blood tests reveal anaemia and a raised ESR. Rheumatoid factor is negative but antinuclear antibodies are positive. The MOST likely diagnosis is

   A acute rheumatic fever
   B juvenile rheumatoid arthritis
   C Still's disease
   D SLE
   E aseptic non-traumatic synovitis

28. The NEXT most appropriate step to guide your further management is

   A echocardiography
   B aspiration of knee joint
   C arrange for MRI scan of the knee
   D arrange for ophthalmology referral for slit-lamp examination
   E blood cultures

29. A 40-year-old man has inadvertently been given adrenaline (epinephrine) IV for anaphylactic shock. He is now in supraventricular tachycardia with a rate of 180/min. Blood pressure is 100/60. Oxygen is administered and vagal manoeuvres are attempted without success. The NEXT most appropriate management would be

   A up to three synchronised DC shocks at 100J: 200J: 360J
   B adenosine 6 mg IV bolus
   C verapamil 5–10 mg IV
   D amiodarone 150 mg IV over 10 min
   E amiodarone 300 mg IV over 1 h

30. Despite your measures, he now complains of chest pain and the rate has increased to 210/min. The most appropriate management NOW would be

   A amiodarone 150 mg IV over 10 min
   B esmolol 40 mg over 1 min followed by infusion at 4 mg/min
   C verapamil 5–10 mg IV
   D digoxin 500 μg IV over 30 min
   E up to three synchronised DC shocks at 100J: 200J: 360J

31. A 60-year-old man collapses on the ward. ECG shows asystole. There is no palpable carotid pulse. The MOST appropriate management is

   A DC cardioversion starting at 200 J
   B 1 min of CPR during which the airway is secured and 1 mg of adrenaline (epinephrine) IV is administered
   C 3 mins of CPR during which the airway is secured and 3 mg of atropine IV is administered
   D repeated precordial blows at a rate of 70/min (percussion pacing)
   E 3 mins of CPR during which the airway is secured and both adrenaline and atropine IV are administered

32. A 70-year-old man presents with calf pain upon exercise, which disappears with rest. He smokes 20 cigarettes a day and takes bendrofluazide for hypertension. He has weak posterior tibial and dorsalis pedis pulses. Ankle-brachial Doppler index is 0.7. All of the following should be considered in his immediate management EXCEPT

A arteriogram
B oxypentifylline
C low dose aspirin
D naftidrofuryl
E stop smoking

33. A 70-year-old man presents with nausea, vomiting and weakness. He has marked peripheral oedema. His medications include digoxin and chlorthalidone for congestive heart failure. Furosemide (frusemide) is administered to which he has marked diuresis of 10 litres and promptly collapses. ECG shows prolonged P-R interval, inverted T waves and depressed ST segments. The MOST likely complication to have occurred is

A transient cardiac arrhythmia
B acute renal failure
C myocardial infarction
D hypoxia
E hypovolaemia

34. A 45-year-old woman presents with severe itching, recent pale stools and dark urine. On examination there is darkened skin pigmentation, xanthelasma and hepatomegaly. Her test results are:

Serum bilirubin   15 μmol/L
Serum alkaline phosphatase   400 IU/L (30–300 IU/L)
AST   40 IU/L (5–35 IU/L)

The MOST likely diagnosis is

A sarcoidosis
B primary biliary cirrhosis
C sclerosing cholangitis
D acute cholecystitis
E common bile duct gallstones

35. A 60-year-old man is brought to casualty unconscious. BP is 60/40, and pulse rate is 35/min. ECG shows Mobitz type II AV block. He does not respond to a total of 3 mg IV of atropine. The DEFINITIVE treatment for this patient is

A transcutaneous pacing
B adrenaline (epinephrine) infusion titrated to response
C transvenous pacing
D synchronised DC shock
E percussion pacing

36. A 30-year-old woman presents with fever and a sharp, constant substernal chest pain. She is clutching her chest and leaning forward in her chair. ECG shows ST-elevation in leads V2-6 and in the limb leads except aVR. Several days later the T-wave inverts in these same leads. The MOST likely diagnosis at presentation is

A post-myocardial infarction syndrome (Dressler's syndrome)
B pulmonary embolism
C coronary artery spasm (Prinzmetal's angina)
D myocardial infarction
E pericarditis

37. Cystic fibrosis is associated with all of the following EXCEPT

A autosomal recessive inheritance
B absent testes
C raised immunoreactive trypsin in affected babies
D deletion of the codon for phenylalanine at position 508 on the long arm of chromosome 7
E nasal polyps

38. Positive end-expiratory pressure ventilation (PEEP) is associated with all of the following EXCEPT

A increased cardiac output
B pneumothorax
C decreased right-to-left shunt
D increased functional residual capacity
E increased arterial oxygen content

39. Extrapulmonary effects of lung carcinoma include all of the following EXCEPT

A syndrome of inappropriate antidiuretic hormone (SIADH)
B carcinoid syndrome
C hypertrophic pulmonary osteoarthropathy
D thrombangiitis obliterans
E Eaton–Lambert syndrome

40. A 50-year-old man complains of dry cough. He is noted to have facial telangiectasias and finger clubbing. On auscultation he has fine-inspiratory crepitations. Chest x-ray shows increased interstitial markings. Lung function tests reveal reduced lung volumes. Bronchoalveolar lavage shows a predominance of neutrophils. The MOST likely diagnosis is

A cryptogenic fibrosing alveolitis
B mesothelioma
C systemic sclerosis
D sarcoidosis
E miliary tuberculosis

41. A 50-year-old obese man presents with headache and drowsiness. He has a history of snoring. He has warm extremities, a flapping tremor and a bounding pulse. On fundoscopic examination papilloedema is present. The MOST likely cause for the papilloedema is

A CO_2 retention (hypercapnia)
B hypoxia
C obstructive sleep apnoea
D cerebral tumour
E malignant hypertension

42. A 25-year-old woman presents to Casualty with light-headedness and breathlessness. She complains of tingling and numbness of her hands. Arterial blood gas:

pH   7.55
$PaCO_2$ 3 kPa
PaO_2 14 kPa
H^+ 25 nmol/L
HCO_3 20 mmol/L

The MOST appropriate management would be

A chest x-ray
B breathe into a paper bag
C activated charcoal
D needle thoracentesis
E V/Q scan

43. A 20-year-old asthmatic presents with increased shortness of breath. On chest examination he is found to have a deviated trachea to the right, reduced tactile fremitus and hyperresonance to percussion on the left. The MOST likely diagnosis is

A right-sided pulmonary embolism
B right-sided pneumothorax
C left-sided pneumothorax
D left bronchopneumonia
E left-sided pleural effusion

44. A 12-year-old boy presents to Casualty with severe dyspnoea. He had been treated by his GP with penicillin for presumed tonsillitis. He uses a salbutamol inhaler for asthma. On examination: temperature 40°C and he is drooling saliva; no trismus. Marked inspiratory stridor and a respiratory rate of 30/min. The MOST appropriate management would be

A oxygen-driven nebuliser
B IV hydrocortisone
C indirect laryngoscopy
D endotracheal intubation under general anaesthesia
E cricothyroidotomy

45. The MOST likely diagnosis is

A croup
B acute epiglottitis
C glandular fever
D acute streptococcal tonsillitis
E acute severe asthma attack

46. A 50-year-old man presents with facial cellulitis. It extends from the front of his forehead down over the bridge of his nose. On fundoscopic examination he has papilloedema. Your MAIN concern is

A meningitis
B cavernous sinus thrombosis
C orbital abscess
D trigeminal herpes zoster
E erysipelas

47. A 50-year-old obese man is brought to Casualty in a confused state. On examination he has nystagmus and is unable to move the eyes fully laterally. He walks with a broad-based gait. He is unaware of his surroundings and grows restless. The MOST appropriate management is

A 50 ml of 50% dextrose IV
B parenteral vitamins B and C (pabrinex) IM
C hydroxocobalamin IM
D oral folic acid
E urgent head CT scan

48. A 40-year-old woman presents with painful eyes and blurred vision. On examination she is found to have a relative afferent pupillary defect and internuclear ophthalmoplegia. On fundoscopic exam there is bilateral papilloedema. Bilateral positive Babinski sign is elicited. The MOST likely diagnosis is

A aneursym of posterior communicating artery (of circle of Willis)
B pontine haemorrhage
C neuromyelitis optica (Devic syndrome)
D SLE
E diabetes mellitus

49. A 30-year-old man presents with a left winged scapula, demonstrated by pushing against a wall with both hands. The nerve that has been affected is

A long thoracic
B dorsal scapular
C suprascapular
D lateral pectoral
E thoracodorsal

50. A 12-year-old girl presents with gradual right hearing loss associated with tinnitus and headache. She denies trauma to the ears and is up-to-date with her immunisations including MMR. The tympanic membrane appears normal. Pure-tone audiogram demonstrates right sensorineural hearing loss. The DEFINITIVE investigation would be

A head CT scan
B MRI of the brain with gadolinium enhancement
C lumbar puncture
D viral titres
E brainstem electric response audiometry

51. The MOST likely diagnosis is

    A herpes zoster oticus (Ramsay–Hunt syndrome)
    B measles virus
    C mumps virus
    D neurofibromatosis type II
    E neurofibromatosis type I

52. A 50-year-old woman presents with bilateral ptosis and diplopia. She has also noticed difficulty in swallowing. All her tendon reflexes are depressed. The MOST likely diagnosis is

    A dystrophia myotonica
    B multiple sclerosis
    C polymyositis
    D myasthenic syndrome (Eaton–Lambert syndrome)
    E myasthenia gravis

53. A 20-year-old woman presents with complete right ptosis. On lifting the eyelid, the eye is seen to be looking down and out. The pupil is dilated. The MOST likely diagnosis is

    A right third nerve and right fourth nerve palsy
    B complete right third nerve palsy
    C incomplete right third nerve palsy
    D Horner's syndrome
    E right third nerve and sixth nerve palsy

54. The MOST common cause of new-onset focal or generalised seizures after the age of 50 is:

    A alcoholism
    B brain abscess
    C brain tumour
    D cerebrovascular disease
    E encephalitis

55. A 40-year-old woman complains of progressive difficulty climbing and descending stairs, rising from a chair or reaching for an object on a top shelf. This has been going on for several months. She has no ocular symptoms but does have mild difficulty swallowing. There is no family history of neurological disorders. On examination her sensation and reflexes are normal. She has some proximal muscle weakness and atrophy. The MOST likely diagnosis is

A myasthenia gravis
B multiple sclerosis
C polymyositis
D motor neurone disease
E myasthenic syndrome (Eaton–Lambert syndrome)

56. A 30-year-old man presents with a right red painful eye. He complains of watering of the eyes and sensitivity to light. He has a history of recurrent cold sores. Fluorescein staining of the cornea demonstrates a tree-shaped sharp-bordered stain. The MOST likely diagnosis is

A dendritic ulcer
B keratoconjunctivitis sicca
C corneal abrasion
D corneal ulcer
E conjunctivitis

57. A 20-year-old woman presents to Casualty with an excruciatingly painful right red eye. She states that her child accidentally poked her in the eye. Her visual acuity and colour vision are both normal. Fluorescein dye confirms a corneal abrasion. The MOST appropriate management would be

A topical application of local anaesthetic
B double eye padding for 48 hours
C refer urgently to ophthalmologist
D arrange for orbital ultrasound
E hypomellose eye lubricant for 2 months

58. The following conditions can mimic panic disorder EXCEPT

A phaeochromocytoma
B hyperthyroidism
C hypoglycaemia
D caffeine withdrawal
E barbiturate withdrawal

59. A 20-year-old man presents for psychotherapy. He is manipulative and lacks empathy. He has a grandiose sense of self-importance and entitlement. The MOST likely personality disorder would be described as

A antisocial
B borderline
C histrionic
D schizotypal
E narcissistic

60. A 22-year-old female presents with secondary amenorrhoea and weight loss. On examination she is noted to have mild parotid swelling. She has a low BP and a body mass index (BMI) of 15. The MOST likely reason for her amenorrhoea is

A prolactinoma
B Addison's disease
C premature ovarian failure
D anorexia nervosa
E bulimia

61. The following are first-rank symptoms of schizophrenia EXCEPT

A anhedonia
B bodily sensations being imposed by an outside agency
C delusional perceptions
D third person auditory hallucinations
E alien thoughts

62. Risk factors for cholelithiasis include all of the following conditions EXCEPT

A Crohn's disease
B haemolytic diseases
C multiparity
D males greater than 40 years of age
E contraceptive pill

63. A 20-year-old woman presents with a temperature of 40°C and a week of bloody diarrhoea. She looks unwell and dehydrated. She has been taking erythromycin for 3 months for acne. She has not travelled abroad, and no one else in the family is unwell. The MOST appropriate management would be

A routine stool culture and microscopy
B admit to hospital, hydrate, take a prompt, direct faecal smear and culture and commence ciprofloxacin
C refer to consultant GI surgeon's outpatient clinic
D admit to hospital, hydrate and request measure *C. difficile* toxin in stool with stool culture and microscopy
E admit to hospital and request urgent GI surgeon consultation

64. Causes of acalculous cholecystitis include all of the following EXCEPT

A Lassa fever
B typhoid fever
C actinomycosis
D scarlet fever
E ascariasis

65. A 50-year-old man presents with weight loss, hiccoughs, jaundice, epigastric and right upper quadrant pain radiating to the back. On examination he is noted to have hepatomegaly, a palpable gallbladder and an abdominal bruit heard in the periumbilical area and left upper quadrant. The MOST likely diagnosis is

A abdominal aortic aneurysm
B gallbladder carcinoma
C hepatocellular carcinoma
D carcinoma of the head of the pancreas
E cholecystitis

66. A 43-year-old man complains of epigastric discomfort, griping widespread abdominal pain and frequent bowel action. There is mucus in the stools. Gastroscopy, abdominal ultrasound, sigmoidoscopy, and barium enema are all normal. The MOST appropriate management would be to give reassurance and

A mebeverine
B diazepam
C metoclopropamide
D omeprazole
E loperamide

67. A 62-year-old woman who has recently undergone liver transplantation for primary biliary cirrhosis presents with pruritis and right upper quadrant tenderness. She has light-coloured stools and dark urine. Her amylase, bilirubin, uric acid, gamma-glutamyl transferase and liver transaminases are all elevated. Her alkaline phosphatase is 2000 IU/L (30–300 IU/L). The MOST likely diagnosis is

A transplant rejection
B common bile duct stricture
C intrahepatic cholestasis
D primary biliary cirrhosis
E carcinoma of the head of the pancreas

68. A 50-year-old man with insulin dependent diabetes mellitus presents with peripheral oedema and ascites. He has 3+ proteinuria. 24-hour urine collection contains 10 g of protein. His serum albumin is 15 g/L. The MOST likely diagnosis is:

A diabetic nephrosclerosis
B nephrotic syndrome
C uraemia
D interstitial nephritis
E retroperitoneal fibrosis

69. An 80-year-old woman presents with chronic dysphagia and weight loss. She complains of a sensation of a lump in her throat, bad breath, and regurgitation of undigested food. She has a history of recurrent chest infections. She does not smoke or drink alcohol. Physical examination reveals a low BMI and a visible lump on the left side of her neck, which is difficult to define on palpation. The MOST definitive investigation would be

A chest x-ray
B barium meal
C endoscopy and biopsy
D oesophageal motility studies
E indirect laryngoscopy

70. A 19-year-old female presents to Casualty with acute onset of right-sided lower quadrant abdominal pain. She states that the pain is getting worse. She last had unprotected sexual intercourse 2 weeks ago. Her period is due today. Blood pressure is 90/50, pulse 100/min and temperature 37°C. On examination the patient has rebound tenderness in both lower quadrants with guarding. Bowel sounds are absent. On pelvic examination there is tenderness on palpating the cervix and right adnexal discomfort. There are no palpable masses. There is blood in the cervical os. The MOST appropriate management would be

A Check urine β-HCG, if positive, resuscitate and crossmatch blood while awaiting urgent gynaecologist referral.
B Take triple swabs and commence broad-spectrum IV antibiotics.
C Resuscitate the patient and refer to surgeons for urgent laparotomy.
D Check urine β-HCG, if positive, send directly to the early pregnancy unit for an urgent transvaginal ultrasound.
E Check urine β-HCG, if positive, arrange for D & C.

71. An 80-year-old man presents with a 2-month history of weakness, dark stools and worsening constipation alternating with episodes of diarrhoea. He has lost a stone in weight. He has a history of diverticular disease and has had two myocardial infarctions. Blood tests reveal anaemia, hyponatraemia, hypokalaemia and hypochloraemia. The stool is positive for occult blood. The MOST useful diagnostic investigation is

A chest and abdomen plain x-rays
B mesenteric angiography
C barium enema
D rigid sigmoidoscopy
E barium swallow and meal

72. The following statements regarding cholesterol are correct EXCEPT

A Cholic acid and chenodeoxycholic acid are derived from cholesterol.
B Gallstones are associated with excessive bile salts in relation to the concentrations of cholesterol and phospholipids.
C The rate limiting step in cholesterol synthesis is HMGCoA reductase.
D Plasma cholesterol is raised in thyroid insufficiency.
E Plasma cholesterol is low in cirrhosis.

73. A 40-year-old woman presents with multiple symptoms. She states that for weeks she has felt tired with a loss of appetite. She has intermittent abdominal pain, diarrhoea and has lost half a stone in weight. On examination: temperature 36.5°C, supine BP is 100/60 with a pulse of 90/min; postural hypotension, mild epigastric pain and a pigmented appendicectomy scar. The BEST test to confirm the likely diagnosis is

A serum urea and electrolytes
B short ACTH (synacthen) stimulation test
C random cortisol
D insulin hypoglycaemia test
E adrenal antibodies

74. A 25-year-old woman a month post-partum presents with a painful diffuse thyroid swelling and fever. Serum thyroxine and ESR are raised. There is no radio-iodine uptake on scanning. The MOST likely diagnosis is

A Hashimoto's disease
B de Quervain's thyroiditis
C Grave's disease
D Reidel's thyroiditis
E multinodular goitre

75. A 30-year-old woman presents with a diffusely enlarged thyroid gland associated with a bruit. Serum thyroxine is raised and TSH is low. The MOST discriminating investigation to establish the aetiology would be

A ultrasound scan
B fine-needle biopsy
C serum thyroid-stimulating immunoglobulins against TSH receptor
D radio-iodine scan
E thyroid releasing hormone (TRH) test

76. A 50-year-old woman is noted to have a high serum calcium, low-normal phosphate and normal albumin on routine biochemistry test. She is asymptomatic. The MOST useful additional blood test would be

A serum chloride
B serum parathyroid hormone (PTH)
C serum magnesium
D serum urea
E serum alkaline phosphatase

77. A 90-year-old man is noted to have a serum alkaline phosphatase of 1050 IU/L (30–300 IU/L) on routine blood tests. He is asymptomatic. Calcium, phosphate and PTH levels are normal. The MOST likely diagnosis is

A multiple myeloma
B osteitis deformans
C bone metastases
D hyperparathyroidism
E osteomalacia

78. A 25-year-old obese lady presents with mood swings, acne, secondary amenorrhoea and hirsutism. She has mild lower back pain, which she relates to her weight problem. She smokes 20 cigarettes a day and drinks alcohol at weekends. BP is 125/85 and urine dipstick is negative for glucose. The MOST discriminating blood test is

A serum LH/ FSH ratio and testosterone
B free T4 and TSH
C serum cortisol
D dexamethasone suppression test
E CEA-125

79. The Multiple Endocrine Neoplasia type I syndrome comprises which ONE of the following

A pituitary adenoma, parathyroid hyperplasia and pancreatic islet cell tumour
B phaeochromocytoma, parathyroid hyperplasia and pancreatic islet cell tumour
C medullary carcinoma of the thyroid, phaeochromocytoma and parathyroid hyperplasia
D phaeochromocytoma, pituitary adenoma and parathyroid hyperplasia
E pituitary adenoma, phaeochromocytoma and pancreatic islet cell tumour

80. A 36-year-old woman diagnosed with premature ovarian failure now presents with bone pain. Serum calcium, phosphate and alkaline phosphatase and urinary calcium are all normal. The MOST likely diagnosis is

A osteomalacia
B osteoporosis
C bone metastasis
D secondary hyperparathyroidism
E multiple myeloma

81. A 50-year-old Middle Eastern woman presents with pain in her thighs. She complains of difficulty in rising from a chair. Serum calcium is low-normal. Serum phosphate is reduced and her alkaline phosphatase is raised. X-ray of her pelvis and femurs show translucent 2-mm bands perpendicular to the surface of the bone extending from the cortex inwards in the right femur. The MOST likely diagnosis is

A osteoporosis
B osteomalacia
C Paget's disease
D polymyalgia rheumatica
E multiple myeloma

82. A 45-year-old female underwent mastectomy with axillary clearance 2 years ago. Following this she developed a manic-depressive illness and now presents with excessive thirst and polyuria. Investigations show:

serum sodium	150 mmol/ L
serum potassium	3.8 mmol/L
serum calcium	3.1 mmol/L
random serum glucose	9 mmol/L
serum urea	6 mmol/L
serum creatinine	100 µmol/L
urine osmolality	150 mosm/kg

Following desmopressin, her urine osmolality increases to 250 mosm/kg. The MOST likely cause for her condition is

A metastatic breast carcinoma
B lithium
C pituitary tumour
D diabetes mellitus
E primary polydipsia

83.

Serum sodium	134 mmol/L	pH	7.20
serum potassium	5.6 mmol/L	pCO$_2$	3 kPa
serum chloride	95 mmol/L		
serum bicarbonate	20 mmol/L		

The above results are ONLY compatible with a diagnosis of

A excessive vomiting
B excessive diarrhoea
C diabetic ketoacidosis
D Addison's disease
E renal tubular disease

84. A 45-year-old woman presents with a 2-month history of fatigue. She smokes 20 cigarettes a day and drinks alcohol at weekends. Her BP is 165/100. Serum AM cortisol is 800 nmol/L (450–700 nmol/L). 24-hour urine collection for urine free cortisol comes back as 1000 nmol/L (<700 nmol/24 hr). Overnight dexamethasone test results in high AM cortisol. However there is some response to high dose dexamethasone. The MOST likely diagnosis is

A ectopic ACTH secretion from small cell carcinoma of the bronchus
B adrenocortical tumour
C Cushing's disease
D alcoholism
E depression

85. A 14-year-old girl with Turner's syndrome presents with short stature. X-rays confirm that the epiphyses have not yet closed. The MOST appropriate management would be

A somatropin
B oestrogen supplementation
C refer for consultation with orthopaedic surgeon for leg-lengthening
D bone scan
E growth hormone levels

86. Causes of transient urinary incontinence include all of the following EXCEPT

A faecal impaction
B atrophic vaginitis
C calcium channel blockers
D tricyclic antidepressant therapy
E delirium

87. Complications of nephrotic syndrome include all of the following EXCEPT

A renal vein thrombosis
B renal artery stenosis
C pneumococcal peritonitis
D hypercholesterolaemia
E hypovolaemia

88. A 30-year-old woman presents with fever, cough and haematuria. She had been in Egypt 2 weeks previously. On examination she has hepatomegaly. Ultrasound shows renal congestion, hydronephrosis and thickened bladder wall but no calcification. The MOST likely diagnosis is

A *Schistosomiasis haematobia*
B *Schistosomiasis mansoni*
C genitourinary tuberculosis
D focal segmental glomerulonephritis
E *Plasmodium malariae*

89. A 30-year-old man presents with acute loin pain and haematuria. He has a history of recurrent urinary tract infections. He states that his father also had kidney problems and had suffered from a bleed in the brain. On examination BP is 160/100, and he has ballotable large, irregular kidneys and hepatomegaly. The MOST definitive investigation would be:

A kidney-ureter-bladder plain film (KUB)
B excretion urography
C CT scan of the abdomen
D renal ultrasound
E urinalysis and MSU for culture and sensitivities

90. Causes of alopecia include all of the following EXCEPT

A zinc deficiency
B iron deficiency
C nicotinic acid (niacin) deficiency
D polycystic ovaries
E pernicious anaemia

91. A 25-year-old man presents with an intensely pruritic rash over his hands, buttock and penis. The itching is worse at night. He had unprotected sexual intercourse a few days ago. On examination there are delicate scaling areas with threadlike linear tracks on the sides of his hands, palms and buttocks. His penis is covered with large, pruritic, crusted papules and nodules. The BEST way to make a diagnosis is

A microscopic examination for mite and eggs on a potassium hydroxide preparation of scraping from tracks
B clear tape removal and microscopic examination for adherent eggs
C VDRL
D skin biopsy with immunofluorescent staining
E direct inspection for multiple eggs and lice

92. Lichen planus lesions are associated with all of the following EXCEPT

A pre-malignancy
B myasthenia gravis
C thiazides
D graft-vs-host disease
E Koebner phenomenon

93. A 20-year-old woman complains of fever, arthralgia and a rash. On examination she is found to have oral aphthous ulcers and pleomorphic erythematous bullous eruptions with concentric rings on her forearms and legs. She is not taking any medication. The MOST likely diagnosis

A erythema multiforme
B erythema nodosum
C erythema marginatum
D pemphigus vulgaris
E Behçet's disease

94. A 30-year-old female presents with a 2-week history of a non-pruritic rash on her trunk, back and upper arms. It started with a single patch on her left scapula. She denies fever or taking medication. On examination she has ovoid erythematous macules with delicate white scaling collars arranged according to the lines of cleavage of the skin. The patch on her left scapula is the largest. Her face, lower arms and lower extremities are spared. The MOST likely cause is

A secondary syphilis
B guttate psoriasis
C nummular eczematous dermatitis
D pityriasis rosea
E erythema chronicum migrans

95. A 30-year-old HIV-positive man on anti-tuberculosis chemotherapy presents with gradual loss of vision in his right eye. On examination he has a relative afferent pupillary defect and loss of red colour vision. The optic disc is slightly swollen. The MOST likely diagnosis is

A TB meningitis
B macular degeneration
C optic neuritis
D CMV retinitis
E optic atrophy

96. A 25-year-old HIV positive man presents with 2 weeks of worsening drowsiness. On examination he has cervical lymphadenopathy and has bilateral upgoing plantar reflexes. CT scan of the head shows cerebral calcifications and ring lesions. The MOST likely diagnosis is

A cerebral toxoplasmosis
B cerebral abscess
C lymphoma
D cryptococcus meningitis
E tuberculosis

97. A 20-year-old woman presents with copious foul-smelling green vaginal discharge and sore throat. She last had unprotected oral and vaginal sexual intercourse 2 days ago. She is 3 months pregnant. The MOST appropriate treatment is

A oral ciprofloxacin 500 mg stat
B oral amoxycillin 3 g stat
C doxycycline 100 mg bd for 5 days
D metronidazole 400 mg tds for 5 days
E cefoxitin 2 g IM + probenecid 1 g by mouth

98. A 22-year-old female presents with frothy gray vaginal discharge. She states that she last had unprotected sexual intercourse 2 weeks ago. The vaginal discharge is noted to have a pH of 5 and emits a fishy odour on alkalinisation with potassium hydroxide. The MOST appropriate treatment is

A oral ciprofloxacin 500 mg stat
B doxycycline 100 mg o bd for 5 days
C metronidazole 400 mg o tds for 5 days
D none as it is not a sexually-transmitted disease
E clotrimazole pessaries

99. A 30-year-old man presents with right ocular pain and blurring of vision and purulent green urethral discharge. He had unprotected sex a week ago. The MOST likely diagnosis is

A chlamydia trachomatis
B Reiter's syndrome
C gonococcal urethritis
D syphilis
E trichomonas

100. A 25-year-old homosexual man presents with swinging fever and rigors. He denies intravenous drug abuse and is not on any medication. On examination he has a pansystolic murmur at the lower sternal border. He is also noted to have pharyngitis and mild proctitis. The MOST likely organism responsible for his presumed infective endocarditis is

A Streptococcus faecalis
B Candida albicans
C Neisseria gonorrhoea
D Streptococcus viridans
E Streptococcus pneumoniae

58/100

Answers to Paper Five BOFs

Criterion Referencing Marks

*   – 25–50% of candidates expected to get correct
**   – 50–75% of candidates expected to get correct
*** – 75–100% of candidates expected to get correct

The notional PASS MARK is 68%

1. E ***

2. E **

3. D **

4. D ***

5. E **

6. B ** The patient has blackwater fever, a complication of infection with P. falciparum.

7. B ** A patient with jaundice and acute renal failure should raise suspicion of leptospirosis (Weil's disease).

8. D *

9. C ** Cryoprecipitate does not contain Factor IX.

10. A ***

11. C ** Blood replacement contains excess citrate associated with hypocalcaemia.

12. E **

13. A * C3a and C5a are chemical mediators of increased vascular permeability.

14. E ** Post-splenectomy may be associated with early thombocytosis.

15. D **

16. B ***

17. B **

18. E ***

19. B ** TCA overdose is associated with fits, arrhythmias, urinary retention and pupillary dilation. Barbiturate poisoning is also associated with pupillary dilation but not with arrhythmias.

20. D ***

21. A **

22. E **

23. C **

24. E * Sodium valproate is associated with inhibition of platelet aggregation and thrombocytopenia.

25. B **

26. D *** This woman most likely has SLE.

27. C **

28. D * The boy's antinuclear antibodies are positive which is associated with the development of iritis and may lead ultimately to blindness.

29. B *

30. E *

31. E *

32. A **

33. A ***

34. B ***

35. C ***

36. E ***

37. B * Cystic fibrosis is associated with absent vas deferens and epididymis.

38. A ** PEEP is associated with decreased cardiac output.

39. D ***

40. A ***

41. A ***

42. B ***

43. C ***

44. D *

45. B *

46. B ** The area of cellulitis in this patient also coincides with the drainage area of the midbrain. Consequently, the patient is at risk of cavernous sinus thrombosis.

47. B ***

48. C ** Devic syndrome is a form of multiple sclerosis.

49. A **

50. B **

51. D ** This patient has bilateral acoustic neuromas.

52. E ** Eaton–Lambert syndrome is associated with small-cell carcinoma of the bronchus.

53. B **

54. D **

55. C ***

56. A ** The cornea stains like a dendritic tree with sharp borders around the ulcer.

57. B ** Topical application of local anaesthetic is contraindicated as the patient will be tempted to rub her eye and extend the corneal abrasion. Double padding is advised to prevent any interference with corneal healing.

58. D ** Caffeine intoxication and not withdrawal may mimic panic disorder.

59. E **

60. D *** Bulimics have irregular periods. Anorexics have no periods.

61. A **

62. D ***

63. D ***

64. A *

65. D **

66. A *** This patient has irritable bowel syndrome which may be treated with an antispasmodic prn.

67. B **

68. B ***

69. B ***

70. A ** The initial management should be to resuscitate the patient and determine whether she is pregnant. Sending a patient in her condition straight up to the early pregnancy unit without IV access and a drip is ill-advised. She will of course require an urgent transvaginal ultrasound to exclude ectopic pregnancy.

71. C ** Colonoscopy, if patient is fit enough, would be the best choice but has not been offered as an option!

72. B **

73. B ***

74. B ***

75. C **

76. B ***

77. B ***

78. A *** This lady most likely has polycystic ovarian syndrome.

79. A **

80. B ***

81. B ***

82. A **

83. C ** The results indicate a metabolic acidosis with an increased anion gap.

84. C ***

85. A * Somatropin is a synthetic human growth hormone produced by recombinant DNA technique and has now replaced somatotrophin (HGH).

86. D ** TCAs have been used to treat urinary incontinence.

87. B ** The patient is at risk of renal vein thrombosis.

88. A **

89. D ***

90. C **

91. A **

92. A **

93. A ** Herpes simplex virus is a common cause of erythema multiforme.

94. D **

95. C * This patient is taking ethambutol as part of his anti-tuberculosis therapy. Ethambutol is associated with optic neuritis.

96. A ***

97. B ***

98. C * Gardnerella is not a STD and usually results from excessive douching and bubble baths but nonetheless is treated with metronidazole for overgrowth of anaerobic bacteria.

99. C *** This patient has iritis and purulent urethritis suggestive of GC.

100. C ***

In these questions candidates must select one answer only

Questions

1. A 20-year-old woman presents with a temperature of 40°C and a week of bloody diarrhoea. She looks unwell and dehydrated. She has been taking erythromycin for 3 months for acne. She has not travelled abroad, and no one else in the family is unwell. Gram-stain of stool show Gram-positive bacilli. The MOST appropriate treatment for her would be

   A IV vancomycin
   B oral metronidazole
   C oral ciprofloxacin
   D oral co-trimoxazole
   E oral chloramphenicol

2. A 20-year-old man back from hitchhiking through South America a fortnight ago now presents with explosive watery foul-smelling diarrhoea and weight loss. On examination he has abdominal distension. His stools are greasy and contain mucus. The MOST likely diagnosis is

   A shigella dysentery
   B giardiasis
   C amoebic dysentery
   D Crohn's disease
   E cystic fibrosis

3. A 24-year-old male living in New England (North-East USA) presents with unilateral facial nerve palsy. He also complains of malaise, neck stiffness, joint pain and a distinctive rash on his leg. The rash started out as a small papule and is now a red ring, 5 cm across with a faded centre. On examination he is also noted to have a pericardial friction rub. The MOST likely diagnosis is

   A Guillain–Barré syndrome
   B sarcoidosis
   C Rocky Mountain spotted fever
   D Lyme disease
   E leprosy

4. The rash is MOST likely

   A erythema marginatum
   B erythema chronicum migrans
   C erythema multiforme
   D erythema nodosum
   E granuloma annulare

5. A 30-year-old 8-week pregnant woman is found to be HIV positive with a viral load of 20,000 and a CD4 count of 300. The MOST appropriate management would be

   A arrange for therapeutic abortion
   B commence therapy with two reverse transcriptase inhibitors (RTI) and one protease inhibitor
   C repeat tests in 3 months
   D commence therapy with two non-nucleoside reverse transcriptase inhibitors (NNRTI) and one protease inhibitor
   E commence therapy with one RTI, one NNRTI and one protease inhibitor

6. A 24-year-old African man presents to Casualty with acute onset of fever, vomiting, jaundice and dark brown-black urine. He had been travelling through Africa 6 weeks ago and had taken chloroquine prophylaxis. He is not taking any medication now. On examination he has irregular fever and BP 100/60. There is hepatosplenomegaly, hypertonia and hyper-reflexia. Serum urea and creatinine are markedly elevated and haemoglobinuria is present. The MOST useful investigation is

   A thin and thick Giemsa-stained blood smears
   B enzyme assay for glucose-6-phosphate dehydrogenase deficiency
   C acid-fast staining of stool
   D hepatitis A, B and C virology
   E yellow fever serology

7. A 30-year-old man presents with cerebellar ataxia a week after eruption of a generalised rash with vesicles. Smear demonstrates multinucleated giant cells. The MOST likely diagnosis is

   A herpes zoster oticus (Ramsay Hunt syndrome)
   B herpes simplex encephalitis
   C varicella zoster
   D tuberculosis
   E neurosyphilis

8. A 30-year-old HIV-positive male presents with seizures. The MOST likely infective cause is

    A toxoplasmosis
    B cytomegalovirus
    C cryptosporidium
    D tuberculosis
    E pneumocystis

9. A 50-year-old female complains of fever, vomiting, abdominal pain and diarrhoea. She dined alone at a restaurant 12 hours ago and had eaten chicken curry and drunk lager and water. Blood tests show:

    serum sodium   134 mmol/L
    serum potassium   2.0 mmol/L
    serum chloride   105 mmol/L
    serum bicarbonate   30 mmol/L

    The BEST immediate management would be

    A admit for IV hydration and IV potassium replacement at 20 mmol/h
    B treat as outpatient with oral fluids, send stool for culture and sensitivities and notify local Public Health Doctor
    C send stool for culture and sensitivities and encourage fluid intake as an outpatient until sensitivities return
    D encourage oral fluid intake and prescribe erythromycin for presumed campylobacter gastroenteritis
    E encourage oral fluid intake and prescribe ciprofloxacin for presumed salmonella gastroenteritis

10. A 50-year-old man with known liver disease presents with fever, abdominal pain and distension. On examination he has a tender abdomen with shifting dullness. Diagnostic aspiration shows elevated neutrophils and Gram-negative rods. The MOST likely organism is

    A *Klebiella* sp.
    B *Escherischia coli*
    C *Pseudomonas aeruginosa*
    D *Bacteriodes fragilis*
    E *Streptococcus pneumoniae*

11. A 20-year-old African male presents with jaundice and acute short-ness of breath. He had been taking primaquine. Blood tests show raised serum bilirubin, reduced serum haptoglobin and anaemia. The blood film shows Heinz bodies and reticulocytosis. He also has haemoglobinuria and increased urinary urobilinogen. The MOST likely diagnosis is

A glucose-6-phosphate dehydrogenase deficiency
B sickle cell anaemia
C paroxysmal nocturnal haemoglobinuria
D pyruvate kinase deficiency
E autoimmune haemolytic anaemia

12. A 35-year-old female presents with a 1-month history of a painless firm but mobile 2-cm lump in the upper outer quadrant of her breast. No other abnormalities detected. The initial investigation should be

A mammogram
B ultrasound
C fine-needle aspiration cytology
D trucut biopsy
E assessment for BRCA1 and 2 mutations with sentinel node biopsy

13. The MOST likely diagnosis is

A breast carcinoma
B fibrocystic disease
C fibroadenoma
D benign mammary dysplasia
E lipoma

14. A 20-year-old female is referred for recurrent epistaxis and bruising. She takes no medication. On examination she has no facial rash or lymphadenopathy. Her spleen is just palpable, and she has generalised bruising but no bone or joint tenderness. Immediate blood test results are

white cell count	5×10^9/L
Hb	10 g/dL
platelets	25×10^9/L
ESR	55 mm/h
MCV	90 fl
MCH	30 pg
MCHC	34 g/dL
prolonged bleeding time	
serum urea	6 mmol/L

The next MOST useful investigation would be

A bone marrow aspirate
B haemoglobin electrophoresis
C platelet autoantibodies
D Factor VIII:C and Factor VIII:vWF assays
E platelet aggregation studies

15. The MOST likely diagnosis is

A thrombotic thrombocytopenic purpura
B idiopathic thrombocytopenic purpura
C aplastic anaemia
D SLE
E von Willebrand's disease

16. A 70-year-old man presents with bruising and bone and joint pain. On examination he has nail splinter haemorrhages. The back of his legs are covered with haemorrhages into the muscles and ecchymoses. X-ray of his legs shows subperiosteal haemorrhages. The MOST likely diagnosis is

A idiopathic thrombocytopenic purpura
B scurvy
C subacute bacterial endocarditis
D aplastic anaemia
E Henoch–Schönlein purpura

17. A 22-year-old female is noted to have both microcyctic and macro-cytic anaemia. She gives a history of intermittent diarrhoea. The MOST likely diagnosis is

A cystic fibrosis
B irritable bowel syndrome
C coeliac disease
D Crohn's disease
E ulcerative colitis

18. A 20-year-old healthy man presents with acute shortness of breath, fullness in the head and blackouts. He smokes 10 cigarettes a day and drinks socially. He is noted to have a ruddy plethora, JVP 6 cm and dilatation of veins on his chest wall. The MOST likely diagnosis is

A bronchial carcinoma
B Hodgkin's lymphoma
C non-Hodgkin's lymphoma
D cor pulmonale
E polycythaemia rubra vera

19. A 20-year-old homosexual man presents with proctalgia and bloody anal discharge. The MOST likely organism would be

A human papilloma virus
B Chlamydia trachomatis
C Neisseria gonorrhoea
D Haemophilus ducreyi
E Treponema pallidum

20. A 45-year-old man on lithium for bipolar disorder is started on ben-drofluazide for recently diagnosed hypertension. The MOST likely complication that might follow is

A decrease in efficacy of lithium
B none as there is no drug interaction
C lithium toxicity
D decrease in efficacy of thiazide
E increased sensitivity to thiazide

21. Heroin withdrawal may be distinguished from cocaine intoxication by which ONE of the following findings?

A pupillary dilation
B hypertension
C sweating
D vomiting
E fever

22. A 36-year-old woman diagnosed with premature ovarian failure now presents with bone pain. Serum calcium, phosphate and alkaline phosphatase and urinary calcium are all normal. Recommended treatment for this patient may include any of the following EXCEPT

A bisphosphonate
B conjugated oestrogen (Premarin)
C raloxifene
D conjugated oestrogen and norgestrel (Prempak)
E calcitonin

23. The following statements regarding calcium are correct EXCEPT

A Calcium and sodium bicarbonate solutions may be administered simultaneously via the same route.
B The initial dose in a patient with tetany is 10 ml of 10% calcium chloride.
C Calcium is not suitable for tracheal administration.
D It is indicated for pulseless electrical activity caused by hyperkalaemia.
E Calcium may precipitate arrhythmias.

24. The following statements regarding fluoxetine are correct EXCEPT

A It is a selective serotonin reuptake inhibitor.
B It is indicated for premenstrual tension.
C It is indicated for bipolar disorder.
D It is indicated for obsessive-compulsive disorder.
E It has some antimuscarinic effects.

25. Which one of the following antiviral drug is LEAST advisable in pregnancy?

A efavirenz
B nelfinavir
C zidovudine
D didanosine
E nevirapine

26. A 20-year-old woman presents with fatigue, nausea, vomiting, and abdominal colic. She has been feeling unwell for many months now living as a squatter in a derelict old house. On examination she is noted to have signs of peripheral neuropathy with a wrist drop. Blood film shows basophilic stippling of red blood cells. The MOST likely diagnosis is

A thalassaemia
B iron poisoning
C lead poisoning
D Crohn's disease
E carbon monoxide poisoning

27. Which one of the following illicit drugs is still detectable in urine for up to 25 days since last used?

A cocaine
B cannabis
C methadone
D heroin
E amphetamine

28. The following are associated with Reiter's syndrome EXCEPT

A keratoderma blenorrhagica
B seropositive polyarticular, asymmetrical arthritis
C painful uveitis
D aortic incompetence
E circinate balanitis

29. A 40-year-old man presents with painful asymmetrical deforming arthritis involving the distal interphalangeal joints and lower back pain. His fingernails are pitted, with onycholysis and linear melanonychia. The MOST likely diagnosis is

A rheumatoid arthritis
B ankylosing spondylitis
C psoriatic arthritis
D osteoarthritis
E inflammatory bowel disease (IBD)

30. A 40-year-old woman presents with fever, symmetrical polyarthralgia affecting the fingers, wrists and knees and weight loss. She is also noted to have alopecia, oral and nasal mucosal ulceration. Full blood count shows anaemia with thrombocytopenia and raised ESR. The MOST definitive investigation is

A rheumatoid factor
B ANA
C anticentromere antibodies
D antibodies to double-stranded DNA
E c-ANCA

31. A 45-year-old woman presents with pruritis and jaundice. She complains of dry eyes and mouth. The MOST discriminating investigation would be

A mitochrondial antibodies
B antinuclear antibody
C serum bilirubin and liver function tests
D HBs antigen
E smooth muscle antibody

32. A 20-year-old man presents with morning back stiffness. He has a history of iritis. On examination he has an early-diastolic murmur. Chest x-ray shows bilateral diffuse reticulonodular shadowing. The MOST likely diagnosis is

A Reiter's syndrome
B Crohn's disease
C rheumatoid arthritis
D ankylosing spondylitis
E sarcoidosis

33. A previously well 55-year-old man presents within 12 hours of the onset of chest pain suggestive of myocardial infarction. ECG shows ST segment elevation greater than 0.2 mV in two adjacent chest leads. The MOST appropriate management would be

A thrombolytic therapy
B IV glycoprotein IIb/ IIIa inhibitor in addition to aspirin and unfractionated heparin
C coronary angiography
D percutaneous transluminal coronary angioplasty
E coronary artery bypass graft

34. A 60-year-old man with a history of angina presents with chest pain. ECG shows ventricular tachycardia. Pulse rate is 200/min, and BP 80/50. Oxygen is applied by face mask. The FIRST action should be

A administer sedation and call urgently for the anaesthetist
B immediate synchronised cardioversion at 100J
C immediate unsynchronised DC cardioversion at 200J
D IV adenosine
E IV lidocaine (lignocaine)

35. A 70-year-old man collapses on the ward. ECG shows ventricular fibrillation. He has a cardiac pacemaker. The minimum distance away from the pacemaker unit for placement of the defibrillator electrodes should be

A 2 cm
B 5 cm
C 8 cm
D 10 cm
E 12 cm

36. Pulseless electrical activity in a cardiac arrest may be associated with all of the following EXCEPT

A tamponade
B thrombo-embolism
C malignant hyperpyrexia
D hypokalaemia
E ruptured aortic aneurysm

37. A 60-year-old man complains of chest pain. 12-lead ECG shows dominant R waves and ST depression in V1-V3. The lesion is MOST likely in the

A left anterior descending coronary artery (LAD)
B diagonal branch of the LAD
C circumflex artery
D right coronary artery
E obtuse marginal branch of the LAD

38. The MOST appropriate management for this patient following oxygen, aspirin, GTN and morphine is

A coronary angiography
B percutaneous transluminal coronary angioplasty (PTCA)
C coronary artery bypass graft
D thrombolytic therapy
E glycoprotein IIb/ IIIa inhibitor and non-fractionated heparin

39. A 50-year-old woman complains of episodes of diplopia and vertigo, worse after exercise. On examination the BP in her right arm is 120/80 and the BP in her left arm is 100/60. A left cervical bruit is noted. The most likely diagnosis is

A coarctation of the aorta
B transient ischaemic attack
C Takayasu's arteritis
D subclavian steal syndrome
E vertebrobasilar insufficiency

40. A 70-year-old man presents with nausea, vomiting and weakness. He has marked peripheral oedema. His medications include digoxin and chlorthalidone for congestive heart failure. Frusemide is administered to which he has marked diuresis of 10 litres and promptly collapses. ECG shows prolonged P-R interval, inverted T waves and depressed ST segments. The MOST useful blood test is

A CK-MB and troponin
B serum urea and electrolytes
C digoxin level
D serum osmolality
E random cortisol

41. A 65-year-old woman presents to Casualty with breathlessness and chest pain. On examination pulse is irregularly irregular and ECG confirms atrial fibrillation at a rate of approximately 180/min. You administer oxygen and gain IV access. The next most appropriate management would be

A heparin and warfarin anticoagulation
B immediate heparin and synchronised DC shock at 100J
C amiodarone 300 mg IV over 1 h
D IV digoxin
E flecainide 100 mg IV over 30 min

42. A 60-year-old man is admitted with congestive heart failure. JVP is 5 cm. Admission bloods are:

white cell count	7×10^9/L
Hb	11 g/dL
platelets	50×10^9/L
MCV	110 fl
MCH	31 pg
MCHC	34 g/dL
AST	45 IU/L (5–35 IU/L)
ALT	50 IU/L (5–35 IU/L)
GGT	190 IU/L (11–51 IU/L)
LDH	300 IU/L (70–250 IU/L)
alk phos	300 IU/L (30–300 IU/L)
serum glucose	5 mmol/L

The MOST likely cause of his congestive heart failure is

A folate deficiency
B vitamin B_{12} deficiency
C haemochromatosis
D alcoholism
E haemolytic anaemia

43. A 20-year-old man complains of high fever, rigors, productive cough with rusty-coloured sputum and pleuritic chest pain. On chest examination he has increased tactile fremitus and dullness to percussion in the right lower lung field. The MOST likely diagnosis is

A lobar pneumonia
B bronchopneumonia
C aspiration pneumonia
D pleural effusion
E lung abscess

44. The drug of first choice is

A cefotaxime
B tetracycline
C erythromycin
D flucloxacillin
E penicillin

45. A 25-year-old woman presents to Casualty with light-headedness and breathlessness. She complains of tingling and numbness of her hands. Arterial blood gas:

pH   7.55
$PaCO_2$ 3 kPa
PaO_2 14 kPa
H+   25 nmol/L
HCO_3 20 mmol/L

The MOST likely diagnosis is

A psychogenic hyperventilation
B salicylate intoxication
C pulmonary oedema
D tension pneumothorax
E pulmonary embolism

46. A 50-year-old obese man presents with headache and drowsiness. He has a history of snoring. He has warm extremities, a flapping tremor and a bounding pulse. On fundoscopic examination papilloedema is present. The MOST appropriate treatment would be

A flumazenil
B doxapram
C naloxone
D hyperbaric oxygen
E diazepam

47. A 50-year-old man presents with dysphagia. On examination he has increased jaw jerk reflex, fasciculation and wasting of the tongue, fasciculation and wasting of the small muscles of the hands and exaggerated lower limb reflexes. No sensory changes are present. The MOST likely diagnosis is

A Parkinson's disease
B multiple sclerosis
C myasthenia gravis
D amyotrophic lateral sclerosis
E pseudobulbar palsy

48. A 50-year-old man presents with progressive dementia over 6 months. His wife states that he is extremely forgetful. He drinks in moderation and smokes 20 cigarettes a day. He takes oxybutinin for urinary incontinence. On neurological examination he has lower extremity spasticity and extensor plantar responses with an ataxic gait. The MOST likely diagnosis is

A thiamine deficiency
B normal pressure hydrocephalus
C Friedreich's ataxia
D Alzheimer's disease
E Huntington's chorea

49. A 60-year-old woman with rheumatoid arthritis presents with neck pain and numbness and tingling in the thumb and first 2 fingers of the right hand. It is worse at night. On examination there is sensory loss in the right hand involving the lateral half of the ring finger and dorsal tips of the first two fingers. The patient is able to flex the interphalangeal joint of the index finger on clasping the hands (Ochner's test). The MOST likely diagnosis is

A complete median nerve lesion
B carpal tunnel syndrome
C median and ulnar nerve palsy
D cervical spondylosis
E cervical rib

50. The MOST useful investigation is

A lateral and antero-posterior cervical-spine x-ray
B MRI scan of the neck
C nerve conduction studies
D hand x-ray
E chest x-ray

51. A 30-year-old female presents with severe headache and vomiting. She is sensitive to light and also complains of neck pain. BP is 170/110 and pulse 50. On examination she has bilateral ptosis, dilated pupils and eyes are positioned down and out. On fundoscopic examination bilateral papilloedema is present. Protein and glucose are present in her urine. Her mental status deteriorates rapidly. The MOST likely diagnosis is

A intracranial tumour
B subdural haematoma
C subarachnoid haemorrhage
D extradural haematoma
E intracerebral haemorrhage

52. Anorexia nervosa may be associated with all of the following EXCEPT

A low white cell count
B low haemoglobin
C low urea
D low bicarbonate
E low potassium

53. A 70-year-old man presents to Casualty after falling when drunk. He complains of sudden numbness and tingling all over both his legs. He also complains of pain between the shoulder blades. On examination he has weakness in his lower extremities, hyperreflexia, positive Babinski, and clonus. The MOST likely diagnosis is

A motor neurone disease
B subacute combined degeneration of the cord
C spinal cord compression
D cauda equina compression
E anterior spinal artery thrombosis

54. A 60-year-old man presents to Casualty with fever and neck pain on passively moving the chin towards the chest. Lumbar puncture shows:

white cells	3000/mm³ predominantly neutrophils
red blood cells	1/ mm³
glucose	1.5 mmol/L
protein	5 g/L

The MOST likely causative organism is

A *Mycobacterium tuberculosis*
B *Neisseria meningitidis*
C *Haemophilus influenzae*
D *Listeria monocytogenes*
E *Streptococcus pneumoniae*

55. A 20-year-old male suffers from ataxia and dysarthria progressing over the past 3 years. On examination he has loss of position sense, lower limb weakness, extensor plantars and absent deep tendon reflexes. He is also noted to have a pes cavus deformity. The MOST likely diagnosis is

A Friedreich's ataxia
B motor neurone disease
C multiple sclerosis
D taboparesis
E peroneal muscular atrophy (Charcot–Marie–Tooth disease)

56. A 40-year-old man presents with diplopia and pain over the left eye. His medication includes lisinopril and Humulin insulin. On examination he has an almost total loss of left eye movement except for sparing lateral and downward eye movementt. His pupils are symmetrical, reactive to light and are of normal size and shape. The MOST likely diagnosis is

A complete III and IV nerve palsy
B mononeuritis involving the III nerve
C complete III nerve palsy
D complete III, IV and VI nerve palsy
E myasthenia gravis

57. A 30-year-old man presents with a right red painful eye. He complains of watering of the eyes and sensitivity to light. He has a history of recurrent cold sores. The most useful investigation is

A slit-lamp examination
B fluorescein dye test
C litmus paper for pH
D Schirmer's test
E smear for Gram-stain

58. A 45-year-old myopic woman comes to Casualty complaining of headache. She states that she also sees flashing lights and cannot see the lower part of objects on the right. Her vision is obscured by what is described as looking through murky water. On examination a field defect is confirmed. The MOST likely diagnosis is

A acute closed angle glaucoma
B uveitis
C migraine with focal aura
D transient ischaemic attack
E retinal detachment

59. A 60-year-old woman presents with sudden painless loss of vision in her right eye. There is no perception of light and there is an afferent pupillary defect. The retina is white with a cherry red spot at the macula. The optic disc is swollen. She is a known hypertensive. The MOST likely diagnosis is

A retinal detachment
B optic neuritis
C central retinal vein occlusion
D ischaemic optic neuropathy
E central retinal artery occlusion

60. A 70-year-old long-sighted woman presented to Casualty at mid-night with vomiting that began three hours earlier and slightly worsening vision. The eyeball fells very hard on palpation. The conjunctiva is injected. The MOST likely diagnosis is

    A acute angle-closure glaucoma
    B anterior uveitis
    C choroidiris
    D retinal vein thrombosis
    E temporal (giant cell) arteritis

61. A 40-year-old woman is referred for psychological assessment. Her latest preoccupation is with the size of her nose, which she believes is too large for her face. She spends several hours a day in front of a mirror. She has had several cosmetic operations to her face, but believes she is still unattractive. On examination her nose looks fine. She is MOST likely suffering from

    A dissociative disorder
    B obsessive compulsive disorder
    C Münchausen's syndrome
    D body dysmorphic disorder
    E somatisation disorder

62. The suicide rate is highest among patients with

    A schizophrenia
    B alcoholism
    C drug addiction
    D borderline personality disorder
    E major affective disorder

63. A 50-year-old obese man is brought to Casualty in a confused state. On examination he has nystagmus and is unable to move the eyes fully laterally. He walks with a broad-based gait. He is unaware of his surroundings and grows restless. The MOST likely diagnosis is

    A subdural haematoma
    B Creutzfeldt–Jakob syndrome
    C Wernicke's encephalopathy
    D Korsakoff's psychosis
    E hypoglycaemia

64. An asymptomatic 60-year-old man is found to have an isolated raised alkaline phosphatase on routine biochemistry. Serum calcium and phosphate levels are normal. The MOST likely diagnosis is

    A osteomalacia
    B multiple myeloma
    C Paget's disease
    D liver metastases
    E hyperparathyroidism

65. The incubation period for hepatitis B is

    A 14–42 days
    B 14–90 days
    C 28–180 days
    D 42–180 days
    E 90–180 days

66. A 62-year-old woman who has recently undergone liver transplantation for primary biliary cirrhosis presents with pruritis and right upper quadrant tenderness. She has light-coloured stools and dark urine. Amylase, bilirubin, uric acid, gamma-glutamyl transferase, transaminases are all elevated. Alkaline phosphatase is 2000 IU/L (30–300 IU/L). The MOST useful initial investigation is

    A abdominal ultrasound
    B percutaneous cholangiogram
    C ERCP
    D liver biopsy
    E abdominal CT scan

67. A 35-year-old female presents with anorexia, fever, abdominal pain, arthralgia and increasing jaundice. She also mentions that she has not had a period for several months. On examination she has acne, hirsuties, bruises, cutaneous striae, hepatosplenomegaly and jaundice. Serum bilirubin, globulin and aminotransferases are high. The MOST likely diagnosis is

    A primary biliary cirrhosis
    B alcoholic Cushing's syndrome
    C Wilson's disease
    D acute viral hepatitis
    E autoimmune chronic active hepatitis

68. An 80-year-old woman presents with dysphagia and weight loss. She complains of a sensation of a lump in her throat, bad breath, and regurgitation of undigested food. She has a history of recurrent chest infections. She does not smoke or drink alcohol. Physical examination reveals a low BMI and a visible lump on the left side of her neck, which is difficult to define on palpation. The MOST likely diagnosis is

A squamous cell carcinoma of the oesophagus
B pharyngeal pouch
C achalasia
D cricopharyngeal spasm
E post-cricoid carcinoma

69. An 80-year-old man presents with a 2-month history of weakness, dark stools and worsening constipation alternating with episodes of diarrhoea. He has lost a stone in weight. He has a history of diverticular disease and has had two myocardial infarctions. Blood tests reveal anaemia, hyponatraemia, hypokalaemia and hypochloraemia. The stool is positive for occult blood. The most likely diagnosis is

A left-sided colonic carcinoma
B right-sided colonic carcinoma
C ischaemic colitis
D diverticulitis
E gastric carcinoma

70. A 28-year-old Jamaican woman presents with acute onset of nausea, vomiting, epigastric pain and ascites. She does not take any medication apart from traditional herbal remedies. On examination she has tender hepatomegaly and profound ascites but no signs of heart failure. She has abnormal liver function tests. The ascitic fluid has high protein content. The investigation of CHOICE is

A isotope scanning of the liver
B hepatic venography
C liver biopsy
D ultrasound scan
E abdominal x-ray

71. The MOST likely diagnosis is

A primary biliary cirrhosis
B hepatic vein thrombosis
C alcoholic hepatitis
D portal vein thrombosis
E Meig's syndrome

72. A 50-year-old woman presents with an abdominal mass and back pain. She denies abdominal pain or abnormal vaginal bleeding having had her last period 9 months ago. Cervical smears have never been abnormal. On examination there is a central mass rising to above the level of the umbilicus. On pelvic examination there is a palpable right adnexal mass. Urine HCG is negative. The MOST useful investigation is

A plain abdominal and lumbar spine x-rays
B CT scan of the abdomen and pelvis
C serum progesterone and β-HCG
D pelvic ultrasound
E CEA-125 tumour marker

73. A 55-year-old man complains of generalised weakness for the past month. He also complains of excessive thirst and frequent micturition. Blood His chest x-ray reveals bilateral hilar lymphadenopathy. The MOST likely diagnosis is

A primary hyperparathyroidism
B sarcoidosis
C lymphoma
D squamous cell bronchial carcinoma
E bone metastases

74. A 60-year-old man presents with sudden severe colicky pain and bloody diarrhoea that began after lunch 3 hours ago. He has a history of two myocardial infarctions. On examination: temperature 39°C, BP 130/90, pulse 110/min regular. There is rebound tenderness in the lower left quadrant of his abdomen and there is fresh blood present in the rectum. There is a raised white cell count and mild anaemia. The MOST likely diagnosis is

A colon carcinoma
B diverticular disease
C inferior mesenteric artery ischaemia
D superior mesenteric artery thromboembolism
E campylobacter infection

75. A 40-year-old woman presents with multiple symptoms. She states that for weeks she has felt tired with a loss of appetite. She has intermittent abdominal pain, diarrhoea and has lost half a stone in weight. On examination: temperature 36.5°C, supine BP 100/60 with a pulse of 90/min; postural hypotension, mild epigastric pain and a pigmented appendicectomy scar. The MOST likely diagnosis is

A hypopituitarism
B diabetes mellitus
C Addison's disease
D hyperthyroidism
E Crohn's disease

76. A 25-year-old obese lady presents with mood swings, acne, secondary amenorrhoea and hirsutism. She has mild lower back pain, which she relates to her weight problem. She smokes 20 cigarettes a day and drinks alcohol at weekends. BP is 125/85 and urine dipstick is negative for glucose. The most likely diagnosis is

A Cushing's syndrome
B polycystic ovary syndrome
C congenital adrenal hyperplasia
D ovarian carcinoma
E hypothyroidism

77. A 90-year-old man is noted to have a serum alkaline phosphatase of 1050 IU/L (30–300 IU/L) on routine blood tests. He is asymptomatic. His calcium, phosphate, and PTH levels are normal. The MOST appropriate management would be

A reassure patient
B abdominal ultrasound scan
C radionucleide bone scan of whole body
D alkaline phosphatase isoenzyme fractionation
E calcium carbonate 1.25 g/vitamin D₃ 400 IU tablets bd

78. A 50-year-old man presents with loss of libido and gynaecomastia. His wife explains that he is always tired and moody. She states that he has physically changed from his holiday photographs. BP is 160/90 and urine dipstick is positive for glucose. The MOST useful investigation to establish the diagnosis is

A thyroid function tests
B short synacthen test
C growth hormone
D testicular ultrasound
E oral glucose tolerance test

79. A 40-year-old woman presents with weight gain and depression. Blood pressure is 150/90 and she has glycosuria. She complains also of secondary amenorrhoea and hirsutism. The most appropriate initial investigations would be

A 24-hour urine collection for urine-free cortisol assay
B overnight dexamethasone suppression test
C serum luteinising hormone and follicle stimulating hormone levels
D serum testosterone
E HbA1C

80. A 16-year-old male presents with gynaecomastia. On examination his arm span exceeds the trunk length and he has small, firm testes. The MOST likely diagnosis is

A testicular feminisation
B congenital adrenal hyperplasia
C Klinefelter's syndrome
D true hermaphroditism
E adrenal 5α-reductase deficiency

81. A 42-year-old woman presents to Casualty with right-sided colicky loin pain and nausea for the past 3 hours. She cannot keep still because of the pain. She has a history of recurrent cystitis. Temperature 36.5°C, BP 110/60 and pulse 60/min. Urinalysis shows microscopic haematuria. While in Casualty the patient develops fever and rigors. The MOST likely complication that has occurred is

A ruptured ectopic pregnancy
B exacerbation of pelvic inflammatory disease
C ruptured appendix
D acute pyelonephritis
E septicaemia

82. A 45-year-old female who underwent mastectomy with axillary clearance 2 years ago now presents with excessive thirst and polyuria. Investigations show:

serum sodium	150 mmol/ L
serum potassium	3.8 mmol/L
serum calcium	2.8 mmol/L
random serum glucose	9 mmol/L
serum urea	6 mmol/L
serum creatinine	100 μmol/L
urine osmolality	150 mosm/kg

The MOST likely diagnosis is

A psychogenic polydipsia
B SIADH
C cranial diabetes insipidus
D metastatic breast cancer
E diabetes mellitus

83. A 50-year-old woman is noted to have a high serum calcium, low-normal phosphate and normal albumin on routine biochemistry test. She is asymptomatic. A subsequent serum parathyroid hormone (PTH) comes back as high. The MOST useful investigation to aid further management is

    A skull, hand, pelvis and chest x-rays
    B ultrasound scan of neck
    C radioisotope thallium/technetium subtraction scan of neck
    D MRI scan of neck
    E CT scan of neck

84. A 60-year-old man presents to Casualty drowsy and confused. Blood test results:

serum sodium	150 mmol/L
serum potassium	5 mmol/L
serum chloride	105 mmol/L
serum bicarbonate	30 mmol/L
serum urea	10 mmol/L
serum glucose	40 mmol/L

    The MOST likely diagnosis is

    A hyperosmolar non-ketotic coma
    B severe diabetic ketoacidosis
    C meningitis
    D encephalitis
    E pre-renal renal failure

85. The following management is advisable EXCEPT

    A 0.9% saline IVI
    B heparin
    C insulin at 3 U/h
    D measure serum potassium hourly
    E blood cultures

86. An 18-year-old known asthmatic presents with severe wheezing and a respiratory rate of 30 and a pulse of 120. She is using her accessory muscles and appears distressed. She is apyrexial. The most appropriate initial management would be

    A IM adrenaline (epinephrine)
    B oxygen and nebulised salbutamol
    C IV dexamethasone
    D endrotracheal intubation
    E IV pencillin

87. A 50-year-old man with insulin dependent diabetes mellitus presents with peripheral oedema and ascites. He has 3+ proteinuria. 24-hour urine collection contains 10 g of protein. His serum albumin is 15 g/L. The MOST effective initial management would be

A oral furosemide (frusemide)
B IV mannitol
C protein restriction
D increase fluid intake
E restrict salt

88. A 30-year-old woman presents with fever, cough, and haematuria. She had been in Egypt 2 weeks prior. On examination she has hepatomegaly. The MOST useful investigation to make the diagnosis is

A IV urogram
B urine for microscopy and culture
C KUB plain film
D cystoscopy
E renal and bladder ultrasound

89. A 35-year-old man presents with progressive weakness in his limbs over the past few days. He had a chest infection 2 weeks prior. On examination he has proximal muscle wasting, hypotonia and absent deep tendon reflexes. His lumbar puncture results are

Cells	4/cc lymphocytes
Chloride	110 mmol/L
Glucose	3.5 mmol/L
Protein	3 g/L

The MOST likely diagnosis is

A poliomyelitis
B botulism
C Guillain–Barré syndrome
D AIDS
E subacute combined degeneration of the cord

90. A 70-year-old man presents with confusion and urinary incontinence. He is pale; BP 160/100. On examination the bladder is palpable to the level of the umbilicus. Rectal examination confirms an
enlarged prostate. There is also peripheral oedema. Blood tests
show:

white cell count	7×10^9/L
Hb	8 g/dL
platelets	100×10^9/L
serum sodium	125 mmol/L
serum potassium	6 mmol/L
serum urea	60 mmol/L
serum calcium	2.4 mmol/L

The working diagnosis is

A chronic renal failure
B acute renal failure
C benign prostatic hypertrophy
D prostate carcinoma
E myelomatosis

91. The MOST appropriate immediate step in management would be

A arrange urgent renal ultrasound
B slow bladder decompression with a sterile catheter
C measure 24 hour urinary protein and creatinine clearance
D arrange urgent IV urogram
E give 10 ml of 10% calcium gluconate and 15 units of insulin with 50 g
   glucose 50% IV

92. The MOST appropriate treatment for moderate acne in an adolescent female is

A erythromycin + topical keratolytic + cyproterone acetate for 3
   months
B benzoyl peroxide 5–10%
C trimethoprim + erythromycin/benzoyl peroxide (Benzamycin)
D retinoic acid
E roaccutane

93. A 70-year-old woman presents with a lesion on her lower right leg,
which has been slowly getting larger over several months. There is a
single scaly flat non-tender red plaque 3 × 4 cm on the lateral side of
her lower leg. It is occasionally itchy. The MOST likely diagnosis is

A squamous cell carcinoma
B psoriasis
C melanoma
D Bowen's disease
E discoid eczema

94. A 20-year-old African female presents with tiny raised spots over her cheeks and neck. The papules are non-tender and non-pruritic but are multiple, scattered and unsightly. The MOST likely diagnosis is

A seborrhoeic warts
B dermatosis papulosa nigra (DPN)
C acne keloidalis nuchae
D molluscum contagiosum
E verruca plana

95. A 25-year-old man presents with an intensely pruritic rash over his hands, buttock and penis. The itching is worse at night. He had unprotected sexual intercourse a few days ago. On examination there are delicate scaling areas with threadlike linear tracks on the sides of his hands, palms and buttocks. His penis is covered with large, pruritic, crusted papules and nodules. The MOST likely diagnosis is

A crab lice
B scabies
C primary syphilis
D jiggers (tungiasis)
E *Enterobius vermicularis* (threadworm)

96. A 60-year-old Mediterranean woman presents with a month's history of rapidly progressive, generalised blistering eruption over her face, chest and axillae. On examination there are randomly scattered tense bullae associated with erosions and crusts. The blisters extend on digital pressure and are easily ruptured and weep. The MOST likely diagnosis is

A pemphigus vulgaris
B bullous pemphigoid
C bullous dermatitis herpetiformis
D erythema multiforme
E bullous impetigo

97. A 50-year-old woman, who is a keen sunbather, presents with a red forehead with a scaly rash. On examination the lesions are multiple, discrete, small, erythematous, with a keratotic surface and varying from a few millimetres to up to 1 cm in diameter; they are gritty to the touch. The MOST appropriate initial management would be

A photodynamic therapy
B metronidazole
C wide excision and graft
D topical fluorouracil (Efudix)
E intradermal triamcinolone

98. A 20-year-old woman presents with copious foul-smelling green vaginal discharge and sore throat. She last had unprotected oral and vaginal sexual intercourse 2 days ago. She is 3 months pregnant. The MOST appropriate management is

A take low vaginal swab for microscopy and culture
B take high vaginal swab for microscopy and culture
C take endocervical swab for virology
D take high vaginal, endocervical and pharyngeal swab for microscopy and culture and endocervical swab for virology
E take low vaginal, high vaginal and endocervical swabs for microscopy and culture and endocervical swab for virology

99. The MOST likely organism is

A *Chlamydia trachomatis*
B *Trichomonas vaginalis*
C *Neisseria gonorrhoea*
D *Gardnerella vaginalis*
E candidiasis

100. A 22-year-old female presents with frothy grey vaginal discharge. She states that she last had unprotected sexual intercourse 2 weeks ago. The vaginal discharge is noted to have a pH of 5 and emits a fishy odour on alkalinisation with potassium hydroxide. The MOST likely organism is

A *Neisseria gonorrhoea*
B *Trichomonas vaginalis*
C candidiasis
D *Chlamydia trachomatis*
E *Gardnerella vaginalis*

Answers to Paper Six BOFs

Criterion Referencing Marks

*   – 25–50% of candidates expected to get correct
**   – 50–75% of candidates expected to get correct
*** – 75–100% of candidates expected to get correct

The notional PASS MARK is 69%

1. B ** This woman most likely has Clostridium difficile infection causing pseudomembranous colitis. Shigella also causes bloody diarrhoea but is not a Gram-positive bacilli.

2. B ***

3. D **

4. B **

5. B *

6. A ***

7. C ***

8. A ***

9. A ** A serum K of <2.5 should be treated with IV potassium replacement. The local Public Health Doctor should be informed regarding a possible food poisoning outbreak from this restaurant.

10. B **

11. A **

12. C ** FNA is less invasive than a trucut biopsy. FNA can also be used to distinguish between a cystic vs a solid lump.

13. C **

14. C **

15. B ***

16. B **

17. C ***

18. B *** In a fit young healthy man think of SVC obstruction as an emergency manifestation of Hodgkin's disease. The treatment is same day radiotherapy.

19. C ***

20. C **

21. E * Fever is present with heroin withdrawal and not with cocaine intoxication.

22. B ** Unopposed oestrogen replacement puts the patient at unnecessary risk for endometrial carcinoma and is ill-advised. Prempak is a form of combined HRT and is a better choice. Raloxifene is licensed for the prevention of vertebral osteoporosis and is a selective oestrogen-receptor modulator.

23. A **

24. C ** Fluoxetine is contraindicated during the manic phase of bipolar disorder.

25. A *

26. C ***

27. B * Cannabis is detectable in urine for up to 27 days with chronic use and for years if a sample of hair is analysed.

28. B *** Reiter's syndrome is a seronegative polyarthritis.

29. C ***

30. D ***

31. A ***

32. D *** Ankylosing spondylitis is associated with both aortic regurgitation and pulmonary fibrosis. X-ray of the spine should show squaring of the vertebrae and a characteristic bamboo spine.

33. A ***

34. A ** The patient needs to be sedated prior to synchronised cardioversion and expert help is required.

35. E *

36. C ** PEA is associated with hypothermia and not hyperthermia.

37. D ** The ECG changes are consistent with a posterior MI.

38. D ***

39. D **

40. B ** Digoxin toxicity may be precipitated by hypokalaemia. The ECG changes are consistent with hypokalaemia.

41. B **

42. D ** The GGT is high and suggests alcoholism as the cause of the macrocytic anaemia and congestive heart failure.

43. A ***

44. E **

45. A ***

46. B **

47. D **

48. B **

49. B **

50. C **

51. C **

52. D ** Anorexia nervosa is associated with a high bicarbonate level due to excessive vomiting.

53. C **

54. E ** *S. pneumoniae* meningitis is more common among the elderly.

55. A **

56. B ** This patient has a partial III palsy as the pupil is spared.

57. B *

58. E **

59. E ***

60. A *

61. D **

62. E **

63. C ***

64. C ***

65. D **

66. A ***

67. E **

68. B ***

69. A ***

70. C ***

71. B ** The patient has veno-occlusive disease secondary to bush tea (Jamaican herbal tea) containing pyrrolidizine alkaloids. This condition resembles Budd–Chiari syndrome.

72. D ** The mass is most likely an ovarian tumour.

73. B ***

74. C **

75. C ***

76. B **

77. A ** As the patient is asymptomatic, no treatment is advised at this time of his likely occult Paget's disease.

78. C **

79. C **

80. C ***

81. D ***

82. C **

83. C ** This investigation is highly diagnostic for parathyroid adenomas and for pre-operative localisation of the parathyroid glands.

84. A *** The anion gap here is 20. Anion gap = (Na + K) − (Cl + HCO3).

85. A ** 0.45% saline should be used if the Na is >150.

86. B ***

87. A ***

88. B ** Suspect schistosomiasis

89. C ***

90. A ***

91. B **

92. A **

93. D **

94. B *

95. B ***

96. A ** Nikolsky's sign is positive when the blisters extend on digital pressure.

97. D ** This is actinic keratosis.

98. D **

99. C ***

100. E **

9/100

In these questions candidates must select one answer only

Questions

1. According to the British Society of Gastroenterology guidelines for dyspepsia, endoscopy is offered to patients with a new onset of dyspepsia and no alarm symptoms lasting for at least 4 weeks who are over the age of

   A 40
   B 45
   C 50
   D 55
   E 60

2. The best confirmatory test for patients with suspected heart failure in lieu of an echocardiogram is

   A beta natriuretic peptide
   B chest x-ray
   C exercise ECG
   D 12-lead ECG
   E troponin C

3. According to the British Thoracic Society Guidelines for the management of stable COPD, the following treatment is advised for a 45-year-old man with breathlessness on exertion, cough and a 39% predicted FEV_1.

   A Regular combined inhaled short-acting beta$_2$ agonists and anticholinergics and 30 mg oral prednisolone for 2 weeks.
   B Regular inhaled short-acting beta$_2$ agonists or regular inhaled anticholinergics and consider corticosteroid therapy if response unsatisfactory after 2 weeks.
   C Regular combined inhaled short-acting beta$_2$ agonists and anticholinergics, corticosteroid trial and antibiotic therapy.
   D Regular inhaled short-acting beta$_2$ agonists and regular inhaled anticholinergics, corticosteroid therapy and long-acting beta$_2$ agonists.
   E Theophylline and long-term oxygen therapy.

4. A 50-year-old Afro-Carribean man requires to start antihypertensive therapy. The SINGLE most appropriate antihypertensive drug based on evidence is

A ACE inhibitor
B angiotensin-II receptor antagonists
C beta-blocker
D calcium antagonist
E thiazide

5. According to evidence-based treatment of metastatic breast carcinoma, the most appropriate treatment option for bony metastases is

A high-dose chemotherapy
B paclitaxel
C radiotherapy
D standard dose chemotherapy
E tamoxifen

6. A 60-year-old man has actinic keratosis of the forehead. He has a history of asthma. The most appropriate treatment is

A camouflage cream
B diclofenac gel
C fluorouracil cream
D intradermal triamcinolone
E tretinoin cream

7. A 60-year-old woman presents with sudden loss of vision in the right eye with acuity reduced to light perception. The retina appears white with a red spot on the macula. She comments that she had transient blindness before full blindness of the right eye. The most likely diagnosis is

A central retinal artery occlusion
B central retinal vein occlusion
C posterior communicating aneurysm
D retinal detachment
E vitreous haemorrhage

8. A 75-year-old man with a history of gout has a persistent BP >170/80 over 3 months. The SINGLE most appropriate antihypertensive drug based on evidence is

A alpha-blocker
B angiotensin-II receptor antagonist
C beta-blocker
D calcium antagonist
E thiazide

9. The ophthalmological side-effect associated with the use of propranolol is

A altered colour vision
B cataract
C diplopia
D dry eyes
E orange-red tears

10. Select the single most appropriate interpretation for the following HBV serology result

sAb +ve   sAg –ve   cAb +ve   eAg –ve   eAb +ve   DNA –ve

A immune, post-vaccination
B immune, past exposure to HBV
C infected, low risk of transmission
D infected, high risk of transmission
E none of the above

11. The Royal College of Physicians Guidelines for Oxygen Therapy recommends use of long-term oxygen therapy after specialist assessment for all of the following conditions EXCEPT

A COPD when Pa_{O_2} <7.3 kPa (on air)
B cystic fibrosis when Pa_{O_2} <7.3 kPa
C obstructive sleep apnoea despite continuous positive airways pressure therapy
D pulmonary hypertension without parenchymal lung involvement when Pa_{O_2} <8 kPa
E pulmonary malignancy with dyspnoea on moderate exertion

12. A 50-year-old heavy smoker presents with a white lesion on the undersurface of his tongue. The SINGLE most likely diagnosis is

A aphthous ulcer
B candidiasis
C leukoplakia
D lichen planus
E ranula

13. A 66-year-old man with Grade III heart failure would benefit from all of the following drugs EXCEPT

    A doxazosin
    B enalapril
    C losartan
    D metoprolol
    E spironolactone

14. Exposure to vinyl chloride is associated with

    A hepatic angiosarcoma
    B hepatocellular carcinoma
    C lung cancer
    D renal failure
    E squamous cell carcinoma of skin

15. Occupational lung allergens include all of the following EXCEPT

    A cadmium
    B colophony
    C fungal α amylase
    D gluteraldehyde
    E isocyanates

16. According to the 2003 British Thoracic Society/SIGN Guidelines on the treatment of asthma, step 3 following introduction of a short-acting beta$_2$-agonist inhaler and regular low dose inhaled steroids is

    A add leukotriene receptor antagonist (LTRA)
    B add long-acting beta$_2$-agonist (LABA)
    C add trial course of oral steroids
    D add SR theophylline
    E double dose of inhaled steroids

17. A 7-year-old boy presents with recurrent abdominal bloating, weight loss and diarrhoea. He is in the 5th percentile for height and weight. The most sensitive screening test is

    A endomysial antibodies
    B full blood count
    C faecal fat estimation
    D serum folate
    E serum vitamin B$_{12}$

18. A 50-year-old woman is noted to have persistently elevated fasting blood glucose. She has a BMI of 31 and has tried unsuccessfully to diet. The most appropriate antidiabetic drug would be

A acarbose
B biguanide
C sulphonylurea
D repaglinide
E thiazolidinedione

19. A 65-year-old lady presents with muscle pains. The full blood count is normal with ESR is 40 mm/h. The next step in management should be

A chest x-ray
B course of high-dose steroids
C reassurance
D temporal artery biopsy
E CRP

20. The mother of an 8-year-old boy would like her son tested for allergy to peanuts as there is a family positive history. Which is the SINGLE most appropriate investigation

A nasal smear
B patch testing
C radioallergosorbent test (RAST)
D serum allergen specific IgE
E skin prick test

21. Risk factors for osteoporosis include all of the following EXCEPT

A gastric surgery
B female gender
C over-exercise
D repeated short courses of steroids
E smoking

22. Diagnosis of diabetes mellitus is best made by

A pancreatic islet cell antibodies
B fasting blood glucose
C HbA1C
D oral glucose tolerance test
E random blood glucose

23. The initial treatment for acute anaphylaxis is

   A 0.5 ml of 1 : 1000 adrenaline (epinephrine) IM
   B 0.5 ml of 1 : 1000 adrenaline IV
   C 0.5 ml of 1 : 1000 adrenaline SC
   D 0.5 ml of 1 : 10 000 adrenaline IM
   E 0.5 ml of 1 : 10 000 adrenaline IV

24. A spirometry result of FEV_1/ FVC = 40% with an FEV_1 of 1.5 L is most likely to be due to

   A asthma
   B extrinsic allergic alveolitis
   C kyphosis
   D sarcoidosis
   E severe emphysema

25. A retrospective study that looks for exposure or presence of a factor association and not causation and which cannot calculate the incidence of a disease but can calculate the odds ratio under certain conditions would be

   A case control
   B cohort
   C cross-sectional
   D randomised controlled
   E snapshot

26. Using the British Hypertension Society 1999 Guidelines for Management of Hypertension, the most appropriate management option for a 55-year-old woman with an initial BP of 170/100 but no cardiovascular complications, diabetes or end-organ damage would be

   A Advise lifestyle changes, confirm within 4–12 weeks and treat if these values are sustained.
   B Advise lifestyle changes, reassess weekly and treat if these values are sustained on repeat measurements over 4–12 weeks.
   C Confirm over 3–4 weeks then treat if these values are sustained.
   D Confirm over 1–2 weeks then treat if these values are sustained.
   E Treat immediately.

27. A study looking at the effectiveness of cognitive behavioural therapy vs antidepressants in the management of phobia is an example of which of the following study designs

    A case-control study
    B cohort study
    C cross-sectional study
    D randomised controlled study
    E none of the above

28. The incidence of DVT in a high-risk population of women aged 35–45 on combined desogestrel and ethinylestradiol is 10%, and the incidence of DVT is 5% in a similar population of women who do not use the combined oral contraceptive pill. The attributable risk is

    A 1%
    B 2%
    C 5%
    D 10%
    E 15%

29. A 70-year-old woman with rheumatoid arthritis presents with rapid onset of multiple mononeuropathies. The most likely diagnosis is

    A Charcot–Marie–Tooth disease
    B chronic symmetrical peripheral neuropathy
    C multiple compression palsies
    D multiple sclerosis
    E multiple vasculitis

30. A 55-year-old man with LV dysfunction continues to have fluid overload and now has sodium retention despite thiazide diuretic, ramipril and bisoprolol. The next drug to add would be

    A amlodipine
    B digoxin
    C furosemide (frusemide)
    D losartan
    E spironolactone

31. If aspirin decreases the risk of cerebrovascular disease by 20%, then the relative risk of cerebrovascular disease in users of aspirin versus nonusers is

    A 0.2
    B 0.4
    C 0.6
    D 0.8
    E 1.2

32. Diagnosis of restrictive cardiomyopathy is made by

    A chest x-ray
    B echocardiogram
    C endomyocardial biopsy
    D ECG
    E MRI scan

33. A 30-year-old woman requests analgaesia for migraine; she is on fluoxetine. The most appropriate form of analgaesia is

    A dispersible aspirin
    B ibuprofen
    C naratriptan
    D paracetamol
    E pizotifen

34. Of the following oral hypoglycaemics the one which stimulates insulin secretion by beta-cells is

    A alpha-glucosidase inhibitors
    B biguanides
    C glitazones
    D guar gum
    E sulphonylureas

35. A 55-year-old man with jaundice is found to have raised plasma conjugated bilirubin and no urinary urobilinogen. The next investigation after viral markers would be

    A CT scan
    B ERCP
    C liver biopsy
    D PTC
    E ultrasound

36. A 50-year-old woman reports headache, nausea, mild eye pain and sees coloured haloes around lights. The most diagnosis is

A cluster headache
B acute iritis
C migraine
D primary angle closure glaucoma
E retinal detachment

37. Select the single most appropriate interpretation for the following HBV serology result

sAb –ve   sAg +ve   cAb +ve   eAg +ve   eAb –ve   DNA +ve

A immune, post vaccination
B immune, past exposure to HBV
C infected, low risk of transmission
D infected, high risk of transmission
E none of the above

38. The following statements are true concerning case control studies EXCEPT

A They cannot calculate risk ratio.
B They are particularly useful for investigating rare diseases.
C They are inexpensive to conduct.
D They can prove causation.
E They are retrospective.

39. Which of the following antihypertensive drugs is NOT correctly matched with its potential side-effect

A alpha-blocker – stress incontinence
B beta-blocker – cold hands and feet
C beta-blocker – impotence
D calcium antagonist – headache
E calcium antagonist – flushing

40. All of the following statements are true concerning anthrax EXCEPT

A Ciprofloxacin is the antibiotic of choice.
B Contacts of exposed individuals do not require prophylaxis.
C Chest x-ray findings are diagnostic.
D ID_{50} is the dose required to infect 50% of exposed individuals.
E It is a notifiable disease.

41. A 26-year-old man presents with a BP of 160/100. Ultrasound shows one kidney is 10 cm in length and the other is 12.5 cm. The most likely cause of this man's hypertension is

A acromegaly
B hyperparathyroidism
C phaeochromocytoma
D polycystic kidney
E renal artery stenosis

42. A 30-year-old woman presents with palpitations. The most useful initial investigation for arrhythmia is

A echocardiogram
B exercise ECG
C 12-lead ECG
D 24-hour-ECG
E 24-hour urinary VMA × 3

43. The SINGLE most common presentation of stroke is

A aphasia
B dysphagia
C loss of consciousness
D sudden onset of hemiplegia
E sudden visual field deficit

44. The following statements are true regarding evidence-based management of stroke EXCEPT

A Aspirin 300 mg should be started within 48 hours of a haemorrhagic stroke.
B Carotid artery stenosis or occlusion is identified by duplex studies.
C DVT and PE develop in 50% of patients after an ischaemic stroke.
D Heparin prophylaxis is indicated if the patient has morbid obesity.
E Heparin is indicated for recurrent embolic TIAs.

45. The SINGLE most appropriate treatment for senile watery rhinorrhoea is

A betamethasone nasal drops
B sympathomimetic drug, i.e. pseudoephedrine
C topical antihistamine nasal spray, i.e. azelastine
D topical nasal ipratropium spray
E cetirizine

46. Initial treatment for allergic nasal polyps as recommended in the BNF is

A beclometasone nasal spray
B betamethasone nasal drops
C oral prednisolone
D sodium cromoglicate nasal spray
E xylometazoline nasal drops

47. The following statements are true concerning renal disease EXCEPT

A Orthostatic proteinuria in an adolescent with a total daily protein excretion of <1 g may be ignored.
B Patients <40 years with microscopic haematuria and hypertension should be referred to a nephrologist.
C Patients with Type 1 diabetes and persistent microalbuminuria should be commenced on an ACE inhibitor.
D Patients with a serum creatinine >150 μmol/L should be referred to a nephrologist.
E Renal function should first be checked 2–3 weeks after initiation of an angiotensin-II receptor inhibitor.

48. The following statements are true concerning drug therapy for obesity EXCEPT

A According to NICE guidelines, patients must have a BMI >30 kg/m^2 and must have achieved a weight loss >2.5 kg over 4 weeks before commencing orlistat.
B Blood pressure and pulse must be monitored frequently prior and during treatment with orlistat.
C Orlistat acts by inhibiting the action of pancreatic lipase thus reducing the digestion and absorption of dietary fat.
D Sibutramine acts by promoting and prolonging satiety after eating.
E Side-effects of orlistat include fatty oily stool.

49. The following studies are correctly matched with their descriptions EXCEPT

A AFCAPS/TexCaps, JAMA – This study showed the benefits of reducing cholesterol in healthy men and women with average cholesterol levels.

B CARE, NEJM 1996 – This randomised controlled trial of 4159 men and women aged 21–75 years who had suffered an MI in the past 2 years and had an average total cholesterol of 5.4 mmol/L were randomised to pravastatin or placebo and followed at 5 years. The study showed that reducing cholesterol level with pravastatin after MI reduced risk of CHD death/non-fatal MI by 24%, of fatal MI by 37% and of stroke by 28%.

C 4S Trial, Lancet 1994 – This was a prospective trial of 4444 patients with coronary heart disease and raised cholesterol. It showed a reduction of relative risk of coronary mortality of 42% in patients treated with simvastatin 20–40 mg a day. Greatest benefit was achieved in patients >60 years of age or patients with DM.

D Heart protection study, Lancet 2002 – This 5-year, randomised controlled study of 20 536 individuals with cardiac disease or diabetes, showed that 40 mg of simvastatin reduced the risk of MI, stroke and revascularisation by one-third, even in patients with normal or low blood cholesterol levels.

E LIPID study, NEJM 1998 – This randomised trial of 6595 middle-aged men with a mean cholesterol of 7 mmol/L showed a 31% reduction in coronary mortality in those treated with 40 mg pravastatin a day and a 20% reduction in cholesterol in the treated group.

50. A 60-year-old woman sensed a 'curtain coming down' over her right eye with painless loss of vision. She mentions seeing flashing lights first. The most likely diagnosis is

A central retinal artery occlusion
B central retinal vein occlusion
C posterior communicating aneurysm
D retinal detachment
E vitreous haemorrhage

51. A 65-year-old woman presents with breathlessness at rest and gross dependent oedema in both legs with breakdown of overlying skin. On examination she has an enlarged tender liver and basal crepitations. The most likely diagnosis is

A cellulitis
B chronic lymphoedema
C congestive heart failure
D deep vein thrombosis
E ruptured Baker's cyst

52. A patient recently commenced on methotrexate for rheumatoid arthritis now complains of a cough. On examination she is afebrile and the chest is clear. The WCC is 11×10^9/L and the platelets are 200×10^9/L. The most appropriate management plan is

A continue current dose of methotrexate
B decrease by 2.5 mg weekly
C discontinue methotrexate
D increase by 2.5 mg weekly
E none of the above

53. A 20-year-old airline stewardess complains of pain in the 3rd and 4th toes. Pain is elicited on compression of the affected web space. The most likely diagnosis is

A arthritis of the subtalar joint
B march fracture
C Morton's metatarsalgia
D plantar fasciitis
E osteochondritis

54. A 70-year-old man with a history of prostatism has a persistent BP >170/100. The SINGLE most appropriate antihypertensive drug based on evidence is

A alpha-blocker
B angiotensin-II receptor antagonist
C beta-blocker
D calcium antagonist
E thiazide

55. A 53-year-old man presents with sharp chest pain. 12-lead ECG shows concave saddle-shaped ST elevation in all leads except aVR. The most likely diagnosis is

A acute myocardial infarction
B acute pericarditis
C aortic aneurysm
D digoxin toxicity
E pulmonary embolus

56. The following statements are true concerning heart failure EXCEPT

A Angiotensin receptor blockers are a first-line therapy in chronic heart failure.
B Beta-blockers are associated with deterioration in the patient's quality of life during the first 3 months of therapy.
C Echocardiogram is the gold standard for diagnosing heart failure.
D NICE recommendations suggest GPs use a blood test for the marker N-terminal pro-brain natriuretic peptide (NT-proBNP) to exclude heart failure.
E Spironolactone should be added to treatment of patients in advanced heart failure (NYHA class III/IV).

57. A 40-year-old man post gastrectomy presents with anaemia. The investigation most likely to reveal the cause is

A ferritin
B folic acid
C full blood count
D vitamin B_{12}
E urea/electrolytes

58. A 30-year-old woman presents with anaemia. She has a history of uterine fibroids. The investigation most likely to reveal the cause is

A bleeding time
B ferritin
C folic acid
D platelets
E prothrombin time

59. A 20-year-old woman presents with recent recurrent epistaxis, easy bruising and heavy periods. The most useful investigation is

A anticardiolipin antibody
B lupus anticoagulant
C platelets
D protein C
E protein S

60. A 35-year-old man presents with chronic fatigue and shortness of breath on mild exertion. He is also noted to have bronzed skin and arthralgia of the MCP joints. The most useful investigation is

A fasting blood glucose
B ferritin
C full blood count
D liver function tests
E rheumatoid factor

61. A 70-year-old man presents with a compression fracture of his spine. The investigation most likely to reveal the diagnosis is

A dexa bone density scan
B full blood count
C serum calcium
D serum protein electrophoresis
E uric acid

62. A 50-year-old man is noted to have stiff joints and swan-neck deformities of his fingers. The most discriminating investigation would be

A antinuclear factor
B ESR
C full blood count
D hand x-ray
E rheumatoid factor

63. According to the NICE guidelines for the management of type 2 diabetes the following statements are true EXCEPT

A Aim for blood pressure below 140/80 mmHg.
B No need to test for microalbuminuria.
C Serum fasting lipids should be measured annually.
D If no manifest cardiovascular disease heart disease risk should be estimated annually.
E If blood pressure >160/100 mmHg should be treated with ACE inhibitors.

64. According to evidence-based medicine, the SINGLE most appropriate step to take in the management of a male patient noted to have a total cholesterol of 6.0 mmol/L, LDL-C 3.5 mmol/L and TG of 2 mmol/L is

A assess coronary heart disease risk
B commence fibrate
C commence statin 40 mg nocte
D offer dietary advice
E refer to specialist lipid clinic

65. A 50-year-old woman reports night sweats and hot flushes. The blood test that would confirm the menopause is

A FSH
B LH
C progesterone
D prolactin
E testosterone

66. The Royal College of Physicians suggest that bone mineral density measurements should be offered to all the following groups of patients EXCEPT

A BMI <19 kg/m^2
B maternal history of hip fracture
C treatment with prednisolone >7.5 mg daily for 6 months or more
D premature menopause (age <45 years)
E radiographic evidence of scoliosis

67. A 9-year-old girl presents with 3 days of fever, sore throat and generalised lymphadenopathy. FBC reveals raised WCC, mostly atypical lymphocytes and mildly elevated ALT. Monospot test comes back as negative. The most appropriate step is

A arrange for immunofluorescence test for EBV-specific IgM
B arrange for liver scan
C repeat monospot test
D reassure patient that she does not have glandular fever
E take throat swab for streptococcus

68. The SINGLE most effective treatment for pseudomonal nail infection is

A calciptriol (Dovonex) scalp application to nails
B gentamicin ear drops
C terbinafine (Lamisil)
D itraconazole (Sporonox)
E topical steroid

69. The SINGLE most effective treatment for palmar hyperhidrosis is

A hydrolloid dressing (DuoDERM)
B topical 5-FU (Efudix)
C paraffin emulsifying ointment (Epaderm), cold tar and salicylic scalp ointment (Cocois)
D intradermal triamcinolone
E iontophoresis

70. Recognised treatment of severe symptomatic pulmonary hypertension includes all of the following EXCEPT

A bosentan (orally active non-selective antagonist of endothelin)
B dobutamine
C heart–lung transplantation
D prostacyclin (epoprostenol) infusion
E regular nebulisation of iloprost

71. The SINGLE most appropriate drug for treatment of depression in the elderly is

A donepezil
B dothiepin
C moclobemide
D sertraline
E venlafaxine

72. A 40-year-old mature student is diagnosed with schizophrenia. His acute psychosis is managed in hospital. Upon discharge, he should be maintained on

A clozapine
B haloperidol
C olanzapine
D pipotiazine
E risperidone

73. A urinanalysis report of RBC 50/mm³, WBC <10/mm³, no organisms, is most likely associated with a diagnosis of

A acute pyelonephritis
B diabetes insipidus
C renal calculus
D renal tuberculosis
E transitional cell carcinoma of the bladder

74. In the treatment of scabies

A It is recommended to wash all bedding in boiling water.
B It is recommended to wash curtains and steam clean carpets.
C It is recommended to take a hot bath prior to application of treatment.
D It is not necessary to treat all the members of a household.
E The treatment should be applied twice, I week apart.

75. A 50-year-old woman with metastatic breast carcinoma complains of unrelenting headaches. The most appropriate analgaesic is

A aspirin
B co-codamol
C diamorphine
D sumatriptan
E tramadol

76. The following statements regarding hypertrophic cardiomyopathy (HOCM) are correct EXCEPT

   A Beta-blockers are used for symptomatic control of HOCM.
   B Children should be screened who have relatives with HOCM.
   C ECG appearance is typical.
   D It is characterised by myocyte disarray on histology.
   E The prevalence in affected families is about 90%.

77. A 70-year-old woman with generalised osteoarthritis presents with stiffness and swelling of the right lower leg and popliteal fossa of the knee. The most likely diagnosis is

   A cellulitis
   B chronic lymphoedema
   C congestive heart failure
   D deep vein thrombosis
   E ruptured Baker's cyst

78. A patient on cisplatin for metastatic seminoma presents with ataxia for several months. He states that his gait is worse in the dark. No other members of his family have similar symptoms, claw toes or pes cavus. On examination the neuropathy is confirmed as sensory. The most likely diagnosis is

   A Charcot–Marie–Tooth disease
   B chronic symmetrical peripheral neuropathy
   C multiple compression palsies
   D multiple sclerosis
   E systemic vasculitis

79. A 30-year-old business man returns from a trip to the Far East and complains of anorexia, malaise, pale stools and dark urine. The SINGLE most useful initial investigation is

   A ERCP
   B liver biopsy
   C liver ultrasound
   D percutaneous transhepatic cholangiography
   E hepatitis viral serology

80. Of the following oral antihypoglycaemics the type which decreases insulin resistance and resensitises the body to its own insulin is

   A alpha-glucosidase inhibitors
   B biguanides
   C glitazones
   D post-prandial glucose regulators
   E sulphonylureas

81. The single most effective treatment for granuloma annulare is

   A hydrocolloid dressing (DuoDERM)
   B topical fluorouracil (Efudix)
   C intradermal triamcinolone
   D prednisolone
   E PUVA

82. An 80-year-old woman requests a laxative for constipation secondary to codeine-containing analgaesia. The following are suitable management options EXCEPT

   A change analgaesia to coproxamol
   B prescribe codanthromer
   C prescribe lactulose
   D prescribe senna
   E suggest increase of fruit and bran in diet

83. A 50-year-old farmer presents with repeated episodes of dry cough, fever and shortness of breath. Chest exam reveals basal crackles. The SINGLE most appropriate treatment option is

   A amoxicillin
   B clarithromycin
   C furosemide (frusemide)
   D prednisolone
   E rifampicin, isoniazid and pyrazinamide

84. The following statements regarding pancreatitis are correct EXCEPT

   A Alcohol and gallstone disease are the main causes of acute pancreatitis in the UK.
   B Cholecystectomy is not recommended at the initial presentation of pancreatitis.
   C Chronic inflammation of the pancreas increases the risk of cancer by a factor of 20.
   D Monitoring of serum CA-19.9 is useful.
   E 20% of patients with gallstone pancreatitis will have a recurrence within 3 months.

85. A 60-year-old man attends A&E with abrupt onset of severe left-sided flank pain. He has a past history of renal colic. He is afebrile. AXR is negative. The urine dipstick is positive for blood and white cells. The next step in management of the patient is

A cystoscopy
B intravenous urography
C spiral CT urography
D ultrasound of kidney, ureter and bladder
E x-ray of spine

86. The following statements regarding hepatitis A are correct EXCEPT

A Alanine aminotransferase levels are markedly elevated.
B Hepatitis A is diagnosed by the presence of IgM antibody to HAV.
C It can give rise to persistent or chronic infection.
D Serum bilirubin is often raised.
E Shellfish is a source of foodbourne HAV infection.

87. The following statements regarding the management of persistent atrial fibrillation (AF) are correct EXCEPT

A Ablation of the AV node and implantation of a permanent pacemaker is a last resort for refractory AF.
B AF is the most common cause of embolic stroke.
C All elderly patients in AF should receive some form of long-term anticoagulation unless contraindicated.
D Calcium channel blockers are the drugs of choice for patients with both AF and coronary heart disease.
E Digoxin may be offered as sole therapy in an elderly, sedentary patient with AF and gastric ulcer.

88. The following statements regarding seizures are correct EXCEPT

A Antiepileptic treatment is not indicated for a single seizure.
B Combination therapy should be employed if seizures continue on initial monotherapy.
C Carbamazepine is the drug of choice for partial-onset seizure.
D Lamotrigine is effective against generalised-onset seizures.
E Twenty years after diagnosis half of patients will have successfully stopped all medication.

89. A 20-year-old man with HIV presents with nephrotic syndrome and hypertension. Renal biopsy shows hyalinisation of glomerular capillaries and positive IF for IgM and C3. The most likely diagnosis is

A focal segmental glomerulosclerosis
B mesangiocapillary glomerulonephritis
C membranous nephropathy
D minimal change glomerulonephritis
E rapidly progressive glomerulonephritis

90. The following statements regarding polymyalgia rheumatica are correct EXCEPT

A Antinuclear antibodies are usually normal.
B ESR is a specific test but is not very sensitive.
C Infliximab may be useful in patients with steroid-resistant PMR.
D Serum interleukin 6 levels are raised.
E Tapering doses of corticosteroids will be required for 2 years.

91. An early sign of retinal detachment is

A coloured haloes
B curtain falling over vision
C flashing lights
D painful loss of vision
E red eye

92. A 31-year-old female with colonic Crohn's disease presents unwell for the third time this year. Her current medication is mesalazine 800 mg tds and azathioprine 150 mg od. She has had two courses of steroids this year. The investigation to assess her known disease is

A barium enema
B CT scan of abdomen
C colonoscopy
D proctoscopy
E flexible sigmoidoscopy

93. Investigation shows mild active disease as far back as the splenic flexure. Blood results are: CRP 50, ESR 39, Hb 11.5 g/dl, with elevated platelets and neutrophils. The most appropriate management is

A change azathioprine to mercaptopurine
B commence oral methotrexate
C commence intravenous metronidazole
D no treatment as she is in remission
E third course of steroids

94. A 40-year-old woman presents with a photosensitive malar rash over both cheeks and the bridge of her nose and chronic musculoskeletal pain. Select the single most discriminating investigation

A anti-neutrophil cytoplasmic antibody
B anti-nuclear antibody
C anti-phospholipid antibody
D antibody to reticulin
E rheumatoid factor

95. The drug of choice for acute pyelonephritis is

A ciprofloxacin
B co-amoxiclavulanic acid
C co-trimoxazole
D nitrofurantoin
E trimethoprim

96. A patient presents with anaemia and an elevated MCV. The following investigations are useful EXCEPT

A ESR
B folate level
C liver function tests
D serum B_{12} level
E thyroid function tests

97. Patients with severe heart failure may benefit from all of the following drugs (unless otherwise contraindicated) EXCEPT

A ACE inhibitor
B beta-blocker
C calcium-channel blocker
D digoxin
E spironolactone

98. Of the following methods the ONE that is NOT recognised for management of scars is

A intralesional corticosteroid injection
B laser therapy
C methotrexate injections
D silicon sheeting
E static splints

99. The single most effective treatment for keloid is

    A hydrocolloid dressing (DuoDERM)
    B topical fluorouracil (Efudix)
    C intradermal triamcinolone
    D self-adhesive silicone gel sheet (Mepiform)
    E cryotherapy

100. The following substances have been shown to cause occupational asthma EXCEPT

    A flour
    B gluteraldehyde
    C isocyanate
    D lead
    E rodent urine

Answers to Paper Seven BOFs

Criterion Referencing Marks

   *   – 25–50% of candidates expected to get correct
  **   – 50–75% of candidates expected to get correct
 ***   – 75–100% of candidates expected to get correct

The notional PASS MARK IS 65%

---

1. D ** The new guidelines advise endoscopy for patients over the age of 55 and not 45.

2. A **

3. A **

4. E ***

5. C ***

6. C * Other treatment options include cryotherapy, surgery or photodynamic therapy. Diclofenac gel may precipitate asthma or hypersensitivity reactions.

7. A **

8. D **

9. D *

10. B **

11. E *** Domiciliary oxygen is recommended for patients with pulmonary embolism or other terminal disease with disabling dyspnoea.

12. C ***

13. A ** The RALES study published in the NEJM in 1999 looked at a large RCT of people with NYHA class III/IV grade of heart failure on treatment including ACE inhibitor and found that adding an aldosterone receptor antagonist (spironolactone) further decreased mortality. The ELITE study published in the Lancet 1997 found that losartan in the elderly reduces symptoms of heart failure and mortality. The CIBIS trial published in the Lancet in 1999 found that long-term use of beta-blockers, i.e. bisoprolol in combination with ACE inhibitors in patients with NYHA class III/IV grade of heart failure, reduced mortality. The SOLVD trial published in the NEJM in 2001 showed that adding enalapril to people on conventional treatment with NYHA class II/III heart failure improves symptoms, reduces mortality and reduces hospital admissions. The MERIT-HF trial, published in the Lancet in 1999, is the largest randomised, double-blind, placebo-controlled, multi-centred study of $beta_1$-blockade in heart failure with 3991 patients treated. The study was conducted in 13 countries in Europe and the USA. This study showed that long-term use of metoprolol CR/XL, in addition to standard therapy including an ACE inhibitor, reduced total mortality and hospitalisation by 31% in people with symptoms compatible with NYHA class II/III.

14. A **

15. A * Cadmium exposure is associated with renal failure.

16. B ** Guidelines have recently been changed as of February 2003. The addition of long-acting $beta_2$ agonists is now advocated, prior to increasing the dose of inhaled steroids to 800 μg/day. If there is no response to an inhaled LABA + increased steroid, then an LTRA or SR theophylline is introduced. Step 4 is, as before, increasing the inhaled steroids to 2000 μg/day and possibly adding an LTRA. Step 5 is the introduction of daily oral steroids.

17. A **

18. B ***

19. C * The upper limits of normal for ESR = (10 + age) divided by 2. This lady's ESR is normal but you may wish to repeat in 6 months. Alarm bells should ring if the ESR was >100 mm/h. Causes of elevated ESR presenting like this include rheumatoid arthritis, infection, malignancy, connective tissue disorders (polymyalgia rheumatica/giant cell arteritis) and sarcoidosis.

20. E ** Skin prick testing should be conducted in a specialist chest clinic as there is a high risk of anaphylaxis.

21. C *** Other risk factors include excessive alcohol, repeated steroid use in inflammatory bowel disease, family history, inactivity, lack of oestrogen and low testosterone in men.

22. B *** A FBG >7 confirms diabetes. If the FBG is borderline (between 7 and 8), do an oral glucose tolerance test. The OGTT should normally be <7.8 at 2 hours postprandial.

23. A ***

24. E *** In obstructive disease, the FEV_1/FVC ratio <80% with an FEV_1 of <80% predicted. In restrictive disease, the FEV_1/FVC ratio >80% with an FEV_1 of <80% predicted. Normally, the FEV_1 should be >80% predicted with an FEV_1/FVC ratio between 70 and 80%.

25. A *

26. B **

27. D ***

28. C * Attributable risk is the incidence in the exposed population minus the incidence in the non-exposed population.

29. E ** Multiple mononeuropathy in a patient with connective tissue disorder is most likely due to vasculitis. Treatment is with steroids ± cyclophosphamide.

30. E **

31. D ** The relative risk in this case is calculated as 1 − (20% of 1) = 0.8.

32. C **

33. C **

34. E ***

35. E ***

36. D **

37. D **

38. D **

39. C ** Impotence is a potential side-effect of thiazide diuretics and angiotensin receptor antagonists.

40. C * Anthrax has an incubation period of 1–7 days. It is a Gram-positive rod diagnosed in cultures from skin or nasal swabs or blood cultures. Three forms of disease include cutaneous (95%), pulmonary and ingestion. Cutaneous anthrax results in a black eschar (malignant pustule) 4–9 days after exposure. Oedema, fever and hepatosplenomegaly may also be present. This form responds to oral ciproflaxacin. Only those directly exposed to spores should be given 60 days of oral ciproflaxacin 500 mg bd. Chest x-ray findings with pulmonary anthrax include widened mediastinum, lymphadenopathy and haemorrhagic mediastinitis. These findings can also occur with tuberculosis. The prognosis is poor.

41. E ***

42. D ***

43. D ***

44. A ** In 2000, the RCP published evidence-based guidelines for the management of stroke. Aspirin should only be started after a CT scan of the head has excluded haemorrhage. Aspirin is indicated for ischaemic stroke. Dipyridamole is offered to patients already on aspirin. Thrombolysis is not routinely offered in the UK, unlike the USA. Heparin prophylaxis is also indicated for prior thromboembolism. In addition heparin is offered to patients with carotid artery dissection. Blood pressure is often high after a stroke and is only treated if it persists. About 75% survive an acute stroke and progress to rehab. Secondary prevention includes smoking cessation, reduction in alcohol and salt intake, mini-dose aspirin and statins if the patient is <75 with evidence of carotid atheroma or h/o CHD. Patients with carotid artery stenosis or occlusion identified by carotid duplex studies, may be offered endarterectomy.

45. D *

46. B *

47. E ** The British Renal Association recommends referral if the serum creatinine is >150 μmol/L. Renal function should be monitored in patients on ACE-I or angiotensin receptor-II inhibitor to exclude renal artery stenosis and should be checked at initiation and 2–3 weeks after any increase in therapy. Many patients with occult atheromatous renal artery disease may end up with renal failure requiring dialysis.

48. B ** Sibutramine requires close monitoring of BP. Orlistat is associated with GI side-effects.

49. E * The 4S or Simvastatin Survival Study was the first trial of LDL-cholesterol lowering with statins for secondary prevention of coronary heart disease.

50. D ***

51. C ***

52. A **

53. C * Pain occurs from pressure on an interdigital neuroma which may require excision.

54. A **

55. B ***

56. A * To reduce pressure on echocardiography services, NICE has implemented guidelines regarding NT-proBNP blood tests for heart failure. ACE inhibitors (i.e. enalapril) and not angiotensin receptor blockers (ARBs) are recommended as first-line therapy for CHF. Renal function must be monitored at the start of treatment and 2–3 weeks following when initiating ACE-I therapy. Loop diuretics are also recommended as first-line therapy. ValHeFT (Valsartan in Heart Failure Trial) showed that ARBs may have a role in CHF in patients who are intolerant to ACE inhibitors and beta-blockers. Beta-blockers show their effect with chronic use and patients should be encouraged to persist with therapy. Use a lower dose in the elderly.

57. A ***

58. B *** This lady most likely has iron-deficiency anaemia secondary to menorrhagia caused by fibroids.

59. C *** This lady most likely has idiopathic thrombocytopenic purpura.

60. B *** This man may have haemochromatosis which is often asymptomatic. Total iron binding capacity and ferritin levels will be raised. LFTs are also deranged.

61. D *** This elderly man may have myeloma, diagnosed by monoclonal globulin spike on serum electrophoresis, plasmacytoma on tissue biopsy or bone marrow plasmacytosis with >30% plasma cells. ESR, calcium and uric acid levels are raised but not diagnostic.

62. E ***

63. B ** NICE guidelines October 2002 now advocate that type 2 diabetic patients also be tested annually for microalbuminuria and if present with a BP >140/80, antihypertensive medication should be commenced. Statins and fibrates should be used to decrease total cholesterol and triglycerides to below 5.0 mmol/L and 3.0 mmol/L respectively.

64. A **Dietary advice should always be offered with advice on lifestyle changes. It is important to assess CHD risk, as this will influence management. CHD risk factors include family history of IHD, smoking, hypertension, diabetes, cerebrovascular or peripheral vascular disease or severe obesity. The British Hyperlipidaemia Association advocate a total cholesterol below 5 mmol/L and triglycerides below 2.3 mmol/L. This patient's fasting lipid results are borderline. Referral to specialist lipid clinics is advised if the total cholesterol level is >7.8 mmol/L or the triglycerides are >4.5 mmol/L (risk of acute pancreatitis).

65. A **An FSH level >30 IU/L with amenorrhoea is diagnostic of the menopause. HRT is now advocated for 2–3 years only and only for the relief of distressing menopausal symptoms. HRT does not offer protection against osteoporosis or heart disease as has been suggested in the past.

66. E **Other risk groups for osteoporosis include patients with thoracic kyphosis, primary hypogonadism, previous fragility fracture, radiographic evidence of osteopenia and chronic disorders associated with osteoporosis.

67. A **In children <10 years of age, only 10% with glandular fever will have a positive monospot test. Also antibodies in glandular fever are transient and peak during the first 2 weeks after clinical onset. So adults may not develop a positive monospot test until a week later. If EBV is strongly suspected in a patient with a negative monospot test, immunofluorescence test is suggested for EBV-specific IgM or EBV serology for anti-EBNA1 IgG.

68. B *

69. E *

70. B *According to the British Heart Foundation, Factfile sheet 01/2003 on pulmonary hypertension, severe symptomatic pulmonary hypertension warrants treatment in its own right. Bosentan is the newest licensed treatment for PPH. Sildenafil (Viagra) is under investigation as a potential form of treatment! There are eight national specialist centres in the UK for the management of pulmonary hypertension.

71. D * SSRIs can be used as first-line therapy although they may be slow to act. TCAs are often used for depression in the elderly but have numerous side-effects – dry mouth, constipation, night sweats, drowsiness, dizziness, vivid dreams and fine tremor. Patients with cardiac arrhythmias on TCAs or who have poorly controlled epilepsy should be offered SSRIs.

72. C * Olanzapine is an atypical antipsychotic without the extrapyramidal side-effects of the older dopamine-blocking drugs. Clozapine is reserved for treatment of refractory schizophrenia and should only be administered in hospital. Depot injections are reserved for patients who are unreliable with oral therapy.

73. E ** Transitional cell carcinoma of the bladder is associated with microscopic haematuria and a sterile pyuria. A patient with microscopic painless haematuria should be referred for urgent cystoscopy.

74. E ** Transmission is through direct skin contact and symptoms result from an immune reaction to the mites' saliva and faeces.

75. E **

76. C *

77. E ***

78. B *** Cisplatin and an underlying neoplasm are both associated with chronic symmetrical peripheral neuropathy. Charcot–Marie–Tooth is autosomal dominant so cannot be included in the differential.

79. E ***

80. C**

81. E *

82. C * Lactulose requires a daily fluid intake of 2 litres or else it will cause severe abdominal cramping and therefore should be avoided in the elderly.

83. D *** This farmer may have extrinsic allergic alveolitis. Treatment is removal of the allergen, oxygen, IV hydrocortisone and oral prednisolone.

84. B **

85. D ** IV urography or spiral CT urography are also options depending upon your hospital's facilities.

86. C ***

87. D ** Beta-blockers and not calcium-channel blockers are the drug of choice here.

88. B* If initial monotherapy is not effective, maximum dose should be used before switching to an alternative choice of monotherapy. Combination therapy is suggested after two failed monotherapies.

89. A * There is a poor response to corticosteroids (10–30%). Cyclophosphamide or ciclosporin may be used.

90. B ** ESR is the most sensitive test but is not specific.

91. C ** It causes painless loss of vision and is an ophthalmological emergency. By the time the patient experiences a 'curtain falling over the vision', it is already late.

92. C *** If colonoscopy is not tolerated, then sigmoidoscopy may indicate disease activity if not extent.

93. E ** The results of both investigations suggest active disease.

94. B *** This lady may have SLE.

95. A ***

96. A ***

97. C ***

98. C * Management of scars may be divided into leave alone, non-invasive and invasive methods. Invasive methods include surgical excision and resuture, resurfacing, peel, dermabrasion, reconstruction with skin grafts, laser therapy, cryotherapy, bleomycin and fluorouracil injections.

99. D * This silicon dressing is now available on NHS prescription and costs £30 for 10 dressings.

100. D **

MRCP Paper Eight BOFs

In these questions candidates must select one answer only

Questions

1. According to randomised controlled trials, the LEAST beneficial treatment for generalised anxiety disorder is

   A alprazolam
   B buspirone
   C cognitive behavioural therapy
   D paroxetine
   E venlafaxine

2. According to evidence-based treatment of metastatic breast carcinoma, first-line therapy for oestrogen-receptor-positive widespread carcinoma is

   A high-dose chemotherapy
   B paclitaxel
   C radiotherapy
   D standard dose chemotherapy
   E tamoxifen

3. A 60-year-old woman with well-controlled BP on ramipril complains of persistent tickly cough. The SINGLE most appropriate replacement antihypertensive drug based on evidence is

   A alpha-blocker
   B angiotensin-II receptor antagonist
   C beta-blocker
   D calcium antagonist
   E thiazide

4. The most effective treatment for scalp ringworm is

   A amphotericin
   B paraffin emulsifying ointment (Epaderm), cold tar and salicylic scalp ointment
   C griseofulvin
   D ketoconazole shampoo
   E selenium sulfide

5. A 15-year-old girl presents with crops of pale erythematous-violaceous macules surrounded by concentric rings on her palms. She had taken a course of penicillin. The most likely diagnosis is

A erythema multiforme
B erythema nodosum
C hand foot and mouth disease
D Kawasaki's disease
E ringworm

6. The one study which is NOT an example of a longitudinal study is

A case control
B cohort
C prevalence
D prospective
E retrospective

7. Factors influencing predicted normal lung function values include all of the following EXCEPT

A age
B ethnic origin
C height
D sex
E weight

8. In the treatment for migraine

A Beta-blockers are useful in the treatment of acute attacks.
B Ergot alkaloids may be prescribed prophylactically.
C Isometheptene mucate in combination with paracetamol is licensed for the treatment of migraines.
D Pizotifen may be used for treatment of acute attacks.
E 5HT$_1$ antagonists are useful in the treatment of acute attacks.

9. A patient's full blood count reveals a low haemoglobin and a normal MCV. The next investigation would be

A assess iron status
B blood film
C reticulocyte count
D ESR
E Hb electrophoresis

10. A 40-year-old woman presents with itching, jaundice and an upper GI bleed. The investigation that is most likely to lead to the underlying diagnosis is

    A anti-mitochondrial antibody
    B anti-neutrophil cytoplasmic antibody
    C anti-nuclear antibody
    D anti-phospholipid antibody
    E antibody to reticulin

11. A patient presents with anaemia and is noted to have spherocytes in a peripheral blood smear. The next investigation is

    A direct Coombs' test
    B reticulocyte count
    C Hb electrophoresis
    D LFTs
    E ultrasound of spleen

12. A patient recently commenced on methotrexate for rheumatoid arthritis reports symptoms only mildly improving. She is still in considerable pain. The WCC is 12×10^9/L and the platelet count is 250×10^9/L. The SINGLE most appropriate management plan is

    A continue current dose of methotrexate
    B decrease by 2.5 mg weekly
    C discontinue methotrexate
    D increase by 2.5 mg weekly
    E none of the above

13. A 30-year-old woman complains of headaches, feeling tired and disorientated. She reports that she recently moved into a council flat, which is damp with visible mould. She also suffers from asthma and is on co-cyprindiol for contraception. The SINGLE most appropriate step in management would be

    A advise patient to test for carbon monoxide poisoning
    B arrange patch testing for mould sensitisation
    C change co-cyprindiol to progestogen-only preparation
    D increase inhalers as the patient is allergic to mould
    E prescribe antidepressant

14. The drug of choice for neuropathic pain is

    A amitriptyline
    B capsaicin
    C carbamazepine
    D gabapentin
    E tramadol

15. A 40-year-old woman presents with a swollen left wrist. She works as a hotel maid. On examination there is swelling over the styloid process of the radius with pain on forced flexion and adduction of the thumb. The SINGLE most likely diagnosis is

A carpal tunnel syndrome
B De Quervain's disease
C Dupuytren's contracture
D scaphoid fracture
E trigger thumb

16. The following statements are correct regarding the 2003 NICE guidelines for the treatment of influenza A or B EXCEPT

A Amantadine should not be used for prophylaxis and treatment of influenza in the same household.
B Oseltamivir is recommended for the treatment of influenza A or B in at-risk patients who can start on treatment within 48 hours of symptom onset.
C Patients with diabetes are included in the at-risk patient group for influenza.
D Zanamivir is recommended for patients over the age of 65 who can start on treatment within 48 hours of symptom onset.
E Zanamivir may be used for the treatment of influenza in patients with hypertension.

17. Regarding smallpox

A According to the Department of Health (DoH), key healthcare personnel across the UK are being offered vaccination.
B Because of the threat of pox virus being used as a terrorist weapon, mass immunisation is needed.
C In the event of an outbreak, the DoH plans to 'contain and ring vaccinate', isolating and vaccinating contacts.
D The smallpox virus has yet to be eradicated.
E Variola virus is an RNA virus.

18. Regarding low back pain

A Lumbar disc prolapse most commonly affects the 30- to 40-year-old age group.
B Lumbar spine x-ray is often useful in the acute setting.
C Patients with concomitant urinary retention should be referred urgently for spinal decompression.
D Surgical discectomy for prolapsed lumbar disc is less effective than chymopapain injections.
E Two weeks bedrest is a first-line treatment option.

19. Regarding MMR vaccination

    A Children with leukaemia are at high risk and should be offered the vaccine.
    B The vaccine is not safe in children who have had an anaphylactic reaction to eggs.
    C The vaccine is associated with autistic enterocollitis.
    D The vaccine contains live, attenuated viruses.
    E. UK recommendations are 1 dose of MMR in childhood.

20. When treating a patient with methotrexate

    A Any profound drop in white cell or platelet count calls for immediate reduction of methotrexate dose.
    B Folinic acid is used to counteract the folate-agonist action of methotrexate and is given 24 hours prior to methotrexate.
    C It is usually prescribed once weekly.
    D It does not cause pneumonitis.
    E Patients require weekly full blood count and renal and liver function tests.

21. Regarding Parkinson's disease

    A Antimuscarinic drugs improve tardive dyskinesia.
    B Levodopa with a dopa-decarboxylase inhibitor is the treatment of choice.
    C Non-smokers have a 60% reduction in risk of Parkinson's disease compared with cigarette smokers.
    D Non-coffee drinkers have a 30% reduction in risk compared with coffee drinkers.
    E Selegeline is not associated with increased mortality.

22. Regarding plantar fasciitis

    A A bony spur projecting forwards from the undersurface of the calcaneal tuberosity is characteristically seen on x-ray.
    B Pain may be elicited on palpation 4 cm anterior to the heel.
    C Patients should be referred to orthopaedic outpatient clinic.
    D Steroid injections are the mainstay of treatment.
    E Stretching exercises to the Achilles tendon are of proven value.

23. The following trials are correctly matched EXCEPT

A MRFIT – This trial showed that increasing blood pressure increases the relative risk of coronary heart disease, stroke and end-stage renal disease.
B DASH – This trial showed that a diet rich in fruit, vegetables, low fat and reduced saturated and total fat can substantially reduce blood pressure.
C SHEP – This trial showed that low-dose diuretic-based treatment is effective in preventing major CVD events, cardiac and cerebral, in both NIDDM and non-diabetic older patients with ischaemic heart disease.
D CAPRIE – This trial showed that aspirin significantly reduced major CV events with the greatest benefit seen in all myocardial infarctions.
E UKPDS – This trial showed that aggressive control of hypertension in diabetics led to a decrease in cardiovascular events.

24. The proportion of true positives correctly identified by the test is called

A absolute risk
B positive predictive value
C relative risk
D sensitivity
E specificity

25. A comparison of case fatalities in patients with diabetes vs non-diabetics following an acute myocardial infarction is an example of which of the following study designs?

A case-control study
B cohort study
C cross-sectional study
D none of the above
E randomised controlled study

26. Using the British Hypertension Society 1999 Guidelines for Management of Hypertension, the most appropriate management option for a 45-year-old man with LVH who is noted to have a BP of 180/105 would be

A Advise lifestyle changes, confirm within 4–12 weeks and treat if these values are sustained.
B Advise lifestyle changes, reassess weekly and treat if these values are sustained on repeat measurements over 4–12 weeks.
C Confirm over 3–4 weeks then treat if these values are sustained.
D Confirm over 1–2 weeks then treat if these values are sustained.
E Treat immediately.

27. A 30-year-old man presents with distal paraesthesiae and distal followed by proximal weakness occurring 1–2 weeks after a GI infection. The reflexes are present initially but become absent within an hour. He soon loses the ability to walk and develops facial and bulbar weakness. The most likely diagnosis is

A Charcot–Marie–Tooth disease
B chronic symmetrical peripheral neuropathy
C Guillain–Barré syndrome
D poliomyelitis
E multiple sclerosis

28. The incidence of DVT in a high-risk population of women aged 35–45 on combined desogestrel and ethinylestradiol is 10%, and the incidence of DVT is 5% in a similar population of women who do not use the combined oral contraceptive pill. The 'numbers needed to treat' is

A 10
B 20
C 25
D 50
E 100

29. A 30-year-old woman is found to have antiphospholipid antibody following a first trimester miscarrage. It is important to exclude

A sarcoidosis
B Sjögren's syndrome
C SLE
D Takayasu's arteritis
E Wegener's granulomatosis

30. A 45-year-old man presents with anorexia and weight loss. On examination he has a palpable, tender liver. Blood tests reveal a polymorph leucocytosis and a prolonged prothrombin time. The MCV is increased. The serum AST and ALT are only mildly elevated. The serum ferritin is 1000 µg/L. The most likely diagnosis is

A alcoholic hepatitis
B drug hepatotoxicity
C liver abscess
D hepatocellular carcinoma
E viral hepatitis

31. A 22-year-old HIV-positive Ugandan man presents with hypopigmented anaesthetic annular lesions with raised erythematous rims and painful nodules on his left forearm and legs. On examination a thickened ulnar nerve is palpated at the left elbow and running into the lesions. He is also noted to have multiple transverse white lines on his fingernails. The MOST useful investigation would be

A complement fixation test
B skin smear for AFB
C biopsy of thickened nerve
D Kveim test
E FTA and VDRL

32. The following statements regarding evidence-based management of breast cancer are correct EXCEPT

A Women with a family history of breast cancer who underwent prophylactic mastectomy have a reduction in death from breast cancer ranging 81 to 94%.
B Prophylactic oophorectomy reduces the risk of breast cancer by approximately 50% in BRCA1 carriers.
C Anastrozole (third-line aromatase inhibitors) is first-line treatment in premenopausal women.
D In postmenopausal women with metastatic disease recurring or progressing on tamoxifen, fulvesterant (selective oestrogen-receptor downregulators) rather than anastrozole was found to be superior.
E Sentinel node biopsy has fewer complications than axillary dissection.

33. A 40-year-old woman is noted to have a 1-cm hard nodule in the upper outer quadrant of her left breast. The biopsy confirms malignancy. The next most appropriate management is

A anastrazole and ovarian ablation
B axillary node clearance and mastectomy
C axillary radiotherapy and mastectomy
D breast-conserving surgery and sentinel node biopsy
E high-dose chemotherapy and tamoxifen

34. If troublesome symptoms persist despite fluid reduction in the evening and cutting out caffeine, men with uncomplicated lower urinary tract symptoms arising from benign enlargement of the prostate should be offered the following treatment for 2–4 weeks

A alpha-blockers
B antimuscarinic drugs
C 5-alpha reductase inhibitors
D referral to urologist
E *Serenoa repens*

35. For acute, generalised pustular psoriasis, psoriatic arthritis, psoriatic erythroderma or for psoriasis not responsive to topical therapy alone, the following treatment should be offered

   A acitretin
   B calcipotriol
   C ciclosporin
   D methotrexate
   E PUVA

36. Which treatment for psoriasis is associated with staining, i.e. of bedding and clothing

   A acitretin
   B calcipotriol
   C coal tar
   D dithranol
   E tazarotene

37. Select the single most appropriate interpretation for the following HBV serology result

   sAb –ve   sAg +ve   cAb +ve   eAg –ve   eAb +ve   DNA –ve

   A immune, post-vaccination
   B immune, past exposure to HBV
   C infected, low risk of transmission
   D infected, high risk of transmission
   E none of the above

38. A 50-year-old man presents with lumbosacral pain without sciatica. The most appropriate management is

   A bedrest and NSAIDs
   B epidural steroid injections
   C exercise and prescribe NSAIDs
   D spine and pelvic x-rays
   E spinal manipulation

39. A tympanic membrane with chalky-white patches is most likely to be associated with

   A cholesteatoma
   B chronic serous otitis media
   C noise-induced hearing loss
   D otosclerosis
   E tympanosclerosis

40. All of the following statements are listed on a patient's steroid card EXCEPT

    A For I year after you stop treatment, you must mention that you have taken steroids.
    B I am a patient on steroid treatment, which must not be stopped suddenly.
    C If you come into contact with chickenpox, see your doctor urgently.
    D If you have taken this medicine for more than 3 weeks, the dose should be reduced gradually when you stop taking steroids unless your doctor says otherwise.
    E If you have never had chickenpox, see your doctor for antibody testing.

41. Select the SINGLE best answer definition of the black triangle symbol in the BNF

    A Denotes those preparations are that considered by the Joint Formulary Committee to be less suitable for prescribing.
    B Identifies newly licensed medicines that are monitored intensively by the MCA/CSM and requires all suspected reactions to be reported through the Yellow Card scheme.
    C Identifies preparations that are not available for NHS prescription.
    D Identifies prescription-only medicines.
    E Requires hand-written requests on FP-10 prescriptions.

42. Extrinsic allergic alveolitis is a form of which type of hypersensitivity reaction?

    A I
    B II
    C III
    D IV
    E V

43. A 50-year-old woman with active rheumatoid arthritis is unable to tolerate both sulfasalazine and methotrexate. She has been on indometacin for the past 3 years. The SINGLE most appropriate alternative treatment is

    A ciclosporin
    B leflunomide
    C misoprostol
    D naproxen
    E rofecoxib

44. A 22-year-old man develops occupational asthma 2 years after starting work in a bakery. The best test to confirm flour allergy is

A chest x-ray
B radioallergosorbent test (RAST)
C patch test
D serum IgG
E skin prick test

45. A 45-year-old woman presents with pain on the underside of the heel. She reports that it is worse first thing in the morning and eases with walking. Walking upstairs makes the pain worse. The most likely diagnosis is

A arthritis of the subtalar joint
B metatarsalgia
C achilles tendonitis
D plantar fasciitis
E postcalcaneal bursitis

46. A 27-year-old marathon runner presents with pain in the shaft of the 2nd metatarsal. X-ray is normal. The most likely diagnosis is

A arthritis of the subtalar joint
B interdigital neuroma
C march fracture
D metatarsalgia
E osteochondritis

47. A 75-year-old woman presents with sudden loss of vision in the left eye with acuity reduced to finger counting. The fundus resembles a bloodstorm! The most likely diagnosis is

A central retinal artery occlusion
B central retinal vein occlusion
C posterior communicating aneurysm
D retinal detachment
E vitreous haemorrhage

48. Of the following antihypertensives the one associated with the rare side-effect of angioedema is

A ACE inhibitor
B angiotensin-II receptor antagonist
C beta-blocker
D calcium-channel blocker
E thiazide diuretic

49. Of the following analgaesics the one associated with elevation of blood pressure is

   A codeine
   B morphine
   C NSAIDs
   D paracetamol
   E none of the above

50. The most common type of malignant thyroid cancer is

   A anaplastic
   B follicular
   C Hurthle cell
   D lymphoma
   E papillary

51. Risk factors for breast cancer include all of the following EXCEPT

   A breastfeeding
   B early menarche
   C first pregnancy >30 years old
   D late menopause
   E nulliparity

52. The following foods are associated with dyspepsia EXCEPT

   A alcohol
   B cucumbers
   C peppermint
   D tomatoes
   E yoghurt

53. Of the following vegetables the one that may affect INR is

   A asparagus
   B aubergine
   C broccoli
   D cucumber
   E lettuce

54. A 65-year-old man presents with right calf pain and swelling. The right leg circumference is greater than the left. He smokes 20 cigarettes a day. The most useful screening investigation is

   A D-dimer assay
   B duplex ultrasonography
   C Homan's sign
   D plethysmography
   E venography

55. The following statements regarding mitral regurgitation are correct EXCEPT

   A Diuretics may relieve symptoms and delay progression.
   B A common cause is dilatation of the mitral annulus secondary to heart failure or left ventricular dilatation.
   C The commonest cause is rheumatic heart disease.
   D The murmur may be mid to late systolic.
   E The murmur may be loudest at the sternum.

56. The following statements regarding arrhythmogenic right ventricular cardiomyopathy (ARVC) are correct EXCEPT

   A About 50% of cases are familial.
   B Histological confirmation of the diagnosis is straightforward and mandatory.
   C It is associated with fibrofatty replacement of the right ventricular myocardium.
   D Sudden death may be the only manifestation of this condition.
   E The treatment of choice for patients successfully resuscitated from a cardiac arrest is an implantable cardioverter defibrillator.

57. If aspirin decreases the risk of cerebrovascular disease by 20%, then the relative risk of cerebrovascular disease in users of aspirin is defined as

   A The incidence of disease in the non-exposed population divided by the incidence of disease in the exposed population.
   B The incidence of disease in the non-exposed population minus the incidence of disease in the exposed population.
   C The incidence of disease in the exposed population divided by the incidence of disease in the non-exposed population.
   D The incidence of disease in the exposed population minus the incidence of disease in the non-exposed population.
   E The incidence of disease in the general population.

58. A 65-year-old woman presents with chronic disabling rheumatoid arthritis. She has a history of peptic ulcer disease and heart failure. The most suitable analgaesic is

A aspirin
B coproxamol
C rofecoxib
D ibuprofen
E prednisolone

59. The following statements regarding pulmonary embolism are correct EXCEPT

A A negative spiral CT excludes clinically significant pulmonary embolism.
B Chest x-ray is often normal.
C It is often associated with high blood pressure.
D Low molecular weight heparins may be used for the early treatment of haemodynamically stable patients.
E Plasma D-dimers have a good negative predictive value.

60. A 60-year-old man presents in heart failure. This is confirmed on chest x-ray. Echocardiogram reveals an ejection fraction of 42% with poor ventricular function and a mildly enlarged left atrium. ECG reveals fast atrial fibrillation. The most appropriate management would be

A Administer thromboprophylaxis prior to cardioversion.
B Cardiovert with amiodarone and add diltiazem to control the rate.
C Cardiovert and control the rate with digoxin.
D Cardiovert and control the rate with timolol.
E DC cardioversion and use verapamil to control the rate.

61. An ECG shows the PR interval is constant, but not all P waves are followed by a QRS complex. The most likely diagnosis is

A first degree heart block
B second degree heart block (Mobitz type I – Wenckebach phenomenon)
C second degree heart block (Mobitz type II)
D third degree heart block
E Wolff–Parkinson–White syndrome

62. The NSF for diabetes has suggested that the ideal target HbA1C should be less than

   A 5%
   B 5.5%
   C 6%
   D 6.5%
   E 7%

63. Of the following oral hypoglycaemics the group which decreases hepatic glucose production is

   A alpha-glucosidase inhibitors
   B biguanides
   C glitazones
   D post-prandial glucose regulators
   E sulphonylureas

64. A 60-year-old woman with metastatic breast cancer asks for analgaesia for headaches. The most appropriate form of analgaesia is

   A diamorphine
   B ibuprofen
   C naratriptan
   D paracetamol
   E tramadol

65. A 45-year-old woman presents with a 3-year history of jaundice, pruritis, pale stools and dark urine. The SINGLE most discriminating investigation is

   A ERCP
   B liver biopsy
   C liver ultrasound
   D serum antimitochondrial antibodies
   E viral serology

66. The most appropriate form of antithrombotic therapy for symptomatic carotid stenosis unfit for surgery is

   A aspirin + dipyridamole
   B simvastatin
   C heparin and angioplasty
   D intra-arterial thrombolysis
   E intravenous heparin

67. The most appropriate form of antithrombotic therapy for intermittent claudication is

A clopidogrel
B aspirin + dipyridamole
C warfarin
D intra-arterial thrombolysis
E intravenous heparin and angioplasty

68. Of the following the one which is NOT a test for female infertility is

A serum FSH taken between days 2 and 5 of menstrual cycle
B serum LH taken 5–10 days before menstruation
C serum progesterone taken 5–10 days prior to menstruation
D serum prolactin
E serum TSH

69. A 60-year-old man presents with recurrent epistaxis, hypertension and microscopic haematuria. The investigation that is most likely to lead to the underlying diagnosis is

A anti-mitochondrial antibody
B anti-neutrophil cytoplasmic antibody
C anti-nuclear antibody
D anti-phospholipid antibody
E antibody to reticulin

70. Maximum predicted heart rate for men is calculated by subtracting the patient's age from

A 200
B 210
C 220
D 230
E 240

71. According to the GMC, chaperones should be offered for all of the following cases EXCEPT

A a female doctor examining a female patient's breasts
B a female doctor performing an abdominal examination on a female patient
C a female doctor performing a PV exam on a female patient
D a female doctor performing a PR exam on a male patient
E a male doctor performing a PR exam on a male patient

72. A 40-year-old woman presents to the outpatient clinic with an acute exacerbation of asthma. Usual peak flow is 390 L/min. Predicted peak flow is 440 L/min. Her peak flow now is 200 L/min. Her current inhalers are salbutamol and fluticasone propionate (Seretide 500). The RR is 20 and pulse 96. On chest examination there are bilateral wheezes and tightness. She has audible wheezes and is breathless at rest. The SINGLE most appropriate initial treatment is

A admit her to hospital
B arrange urgent chest x-ray
C prescribe a volumatic spacer and instruct her to put 12 puffs of salbutamol into the spacer and inhale
D prescribe a week's course of amoxicillin and prednisolone
E start nebuliser treatment with salbutamol and ipratropium

73. A 45-year-old patient with NIDDM on metformin continues to have a HbA1C of 9 for 6 months despite drug compliance. The BMI is 30. According to evidence-based medicine, the SINGLE most appropriate step is to

A add acarbose
B add glitazone
C change to sulphonylurea
D convert to insulin therapy
E add sibutramine

74. A 16-year-old girl presents with mild acne vulgaris. The single most appropriate treatment is

A benzoyl peroxide
B co-cyprindiol
C isotretinoin
D oral doxycycline
E oxytetracycline

75. The following statements regarding acute cholecystitis are correct EXCEPT

A Delayed or 'interval' surgery is preferable to early cholecystectomy.
B First-line treatment includes nil by mouth, IV fluids and analgaesia.
C It is most often caused by gallstones.
D Patients suspected of having acute cholecystitis should be referred to hospital immediately.
E Percutaneous cholecystostomy is a safe alternative to cholecystectomy for those unfit for a general anaesthetic.

76. The following statements regarding treatment of generalised anxiety disorder are correct EXCEPT

    A Benzodiazepines have been implicated in up to 10% of road traffic accidents.
    B Buspirone improves symptoms in the long term.
    C Cognitive therapy focuses on patients' current problems and not their past.
    D The best treatment is cognitive therapy
    E There is no significant difference between paroxetine and venlafaxine in reducing symptoms in the short term.

77. Presenting symptoms of head and neck cancer include all of the following EXCEPT

    A cervicalgia
    B cervical lymph node enlargement
    C dysphagia
    D earache
    E hoarseness

78. A 20-year-old heavy smoker reports spells of headaches lasting 2–3 months each year. He has pain around his left eye, mostly at night. He has to bang his head against the wall, as the pain is intolerable. The pain lasts for an hour. On examination the eye is red and watering with blocked nose. The most likely diagnosis is

    A cluster headache
    B idiopathic intracranial hypertension
    C intracranial tumour
    D migraine
    E primary angle closure glaucoma

79. A 60-year-old man with jaundice is noted to have dilation of the common bile duct on ultrasonography but a normal PTC. The next step in management would be

    A CT scan
    B ERCP
    C liver biopsy
    D liver isotope scan
    E repeat ultrasound

80. A 60-year-old woman on ramipril develops a tickly cough. Chest examination is normal. After stopping the drug the next best treatment is

    A amoxicillin
    B beclometasone nasal spray
    C losartan
    D prednisolone
    E salbutamol inhaler

81. The following are suggestive of Addison's disease EXCEPT

    A hyponatraemia
    B hypokalaemia
    C loss of axillary hair
    D postural hypotension
    E palmar pigmentation

82. The SINGLE preferred imaging method to distinguish Parkinson's disease from essential tremor is

    A CT scan
    B FP-CIT (DaTSCAN)
    C magnetoencephalography
    D MRI scan
    E MR spectroscopy

83. High 'pathological' myopia is a risk factor for all of the following eye conditions EXCEPT

    A central retinal vein occlusion
    B glaucoma
    C macular degeneration
    D retinal detachment
    E strabismus

84. A 60-year-old obese woman presents with non-pitting oedema in both lower legs some weeks following bilateral knee replacement. The most likely diagnosis is

    A cellulitis
    B chronic lymphoedema
    C congestive heart failure
    D deep vein thrombosis
    E ruptured Baker's cysts

85. A 40-year-old man complained of a painful red eye with photophobia and pain on accommodation. The pupil is irregular. The most likely diagnosis is

A acute conjunctivitis
B acute iritis
C central retinal artery occlusion
D central retinal vein occlusion
E retinal detachment

86. A 40-year-old carpenter presents with pain on the lateral aspect of his elbow. He reports that the pain is worse when he uses a screwdriver. He has tried NSAIDs with no relief of symptoms. The next most appropriate form of analgaesia is

A co-codamol
B co-proxamol
C paracetamol
D local steroid injection
E tramadol

87. Bulimia may be associated with all of the following EXCEPT

A binge drinking
B bipolar disorder
C normal weight
D score lines on the backs of the hands (Russell's sign)
E swollen parotid glands

88. A 40-year-old woman presents with severe renal colic. The SINGLE most appropriate form of analgaesia (unless contraindicated) is

A IM diclofenac
B IM morphine sulphate and cyclizine
C IM pethidine
D oral morphine
E rectal diclofenac

89. Risk factors for obstructive sleep apnoea include all of the following EXCEPT

A bifid uvula
B genetic predisposition
C obesity
D redundant uvula
E smoking

90. A 60-year-old woman presents with bruising. She has a recent history of gout. On examination, the spleen is palpable. The white cell and platelet counts are both elevated, and there is an increase in red blood cell mass. The SINGLE most likely diagnosis is

    A chronic myeloid leukaemia
    B essential thrombocythaemia
    C multiple myeloma
    D polycythaemia rubra vera
    E primary myelosclerosis

91. The SINGLE best treatment is

    A busulfan
    B hydroxyurea
    C melphalan
    D supportive
    E venesection

92. A 40-year-old man complains of shoulder pain. On examination he has pain when abducting his shoulder from 45 degrees below the horizontal to 45 degrees above. Pain is also elicited on pushing down on his raised arm. The SINGLE most likely diagnosis is

    A adhesive capsulitis
    B cervical spondylosis
    C glenohumeral subluxation
    D injury of the spinal accessory nerve
    E rotator cuff tendonitis

93. Psoriasis may be exacerbated by all of the following factors EXCEPT

    A alcohol
    B beta-blockers
    C NSAIDs
    D sunlight
    E tonsillitis treated with antibiotics

94. The single most effective treatment for lamellar splitting of the nails is

    A calcipotriol (Dovonex) scalp solution on nails
    B gloves and moisturiser
    C terbinafine (Lamisil)
    D itraconazole (Sporanox)
    E topical steroid

95. A 50-year-old homeless man smelling of alcohol presents with fever and a productive cough. Chest exam reveals coarse rhonchi. The best treatment is

A amoxicillin
B clarithromycin
C gentamicin
D prednisolone
E rifampicin, isoniazid and pyrazinamide

96. A 66-year-old woman is noted to have developed kyphosis. The most appropriate management would be

A arrange a dexa scan
B arrange a thoracic spine x-ray
C commence alendronate
D start on daily calcichew forte
E take blood for calcium and phosphate levels

97. The single most effective treatment for psoriasis of the nails is

A calciptriol (Dovonex) scalp application to nails
B gentamicin ear drops
C terbinafine (Lamisil)
D itraconazole (Sporanox)
E topical steroid

98. A 55-year-old man with COPD is noted to have a unilateral wheeze on chest auscultation. The most likely diagnosis is

A chest infection
B exacerabation of COPD
C lung carcinoma
D pulmonary embolus
E pulmonary fibrosis

99. A 40-year-old man presents with jaundice and malaise. His ferritin level is high and his LFTs are mildly elevated. He does not drink alcohol. The SINGLE most discriminating investigation is

A ERCP
B liver biopsy
C liver ultrasound
D percutaneous transhepatic cholangiography
E viral serology

100. Exceptions to generic prescribing include all of the following EXCEPT

A theophylline
B ciclosporin
C diltiazem
D losartan
E nifedipine

Answers to Paper Eight BOFs

Criterion Referencing Marks

*   – 25–50% of candidates expected to get correct
**   – 50–75% of candidates expected to get correct
***   – 75–100% of candidates expected to get correct

The notional PASS MARK is 59%

1. A *

2. E **

3. B **

4. C * Epaderm and Cocois is the treatment for pityriasis capitis. Epaderm is a soap substitute and is applied overnight to the scalp and washed out to descale the scalp. Then Cocois should be applied in half-inch intervals. Topical treatment is ineffective in scalp ringworm. Scrapings should be taken and oral griseofulvin or oral terbinafine commenced.

5. A ***

6. C **

7. E *

8. C * Serotonin agonists, i.e. sumatriptan, naratriptan and rizatriptan, are used for the treatment of acute attacks. Ergot alkaloids should never be used prophylactically, as they are associated with many side-effects – GI upset and muscle cramps. Pizotifen is useful for the prevention of migraines. Beta-blockers may be used in migraine prophylaxis.

9. B ***

10. A *** This lady may have primary biliary cirrhosis.

11. B ***

12. D **

13. A * The flat may not have central heating and if the walls are mouldy, then concern arises as to whether there is a gas leak from poor gas maintenance also.

14. A ** Starting dose of amitripytiline should be 10 mg nocte and increased slowly up to 75 mg if necessary. Carabamazepine and gabapentin are second-line drugs. Tramadol is used for nociceptive pain. Topical capsaicin has been used for neuropathic pain but some patients cannot tolerate the initial increase in pain.

15. B * Pain on forced flexion and adduction of the thumb is a positive Finckelstein's sign for De Quervain's tenosynovitis (stenosing tenovaginitis). The cause of the condition is unknown; however wringing motion of the hands, i.e. drying out clothes, aggravates the condition. Treatment may involve steroid injection around the tendons or surgical decompression.

16. E * Both oseltamivir and zanamivir have been approved by NICE in 2003 for the treatment of adults at risk of influenza A or B who can start on treatment within 48 hours of symptom onset. Oseltamivir is recommended for children who are at risk. At-risk categories include patients over the age of 65, patients with COPD or asthma, DM, significant CV disease (excluding hypertension) or those with immunosuppression.

17. A ** The DoH plans to offer vaccination to 350 key healthcare personnel across the UK (12 Smallpox Response Groups established around the UK) who would provide the first response in the event of a confirmed, suspected or threatened release of smallpox (a DNA pox virus). The smallpox virus was certified by the World Health Organisation as eradicated in 1979.

18. C *** Prolapsed lumbar disc is most common in the 20- to 30-year-old age group. The discs involved are L4/5 or L5/S1. 90% of patients are better within 6 weeks and 95% by 3 months. Gentle early mobilisation and physiotherapy with analgaesia is advocated. The Cochrane review from 2001 concluded that bedrest was not effective and may be deleterious. Surgical discectomy is much more effective than chymopapain injections for prolapsed lumbar disc.

19. D * The UK recommends 2 doses of MMR in childhood.

20. C * Methotrexate-induced pneumonitis is treated with corticosteroids. The Committee on Safety of Medicines has recommended a new warning label on methotrexate after numerous medication errors and overdosing. Methotrexate is usually given once weekly for the treatment of leukaemia, psoriasis and rheumatic disease. Folic acid is given once weekly after the dose of methotrexate to counteract the folate-antagonist effect of methotrexate. Blood tests are recommended before treatment commences and weekly until therapy stabilises. Thereafter patients should be monitored every 2–3 months. Any drastic drop in white cell or platelet count calls for immediate withdrawal of methotrexate and administration of supportive therapy.

21. B ** Nicotine and caffeine have been proven to play a protective role in the development of Parkinson's disease. Antimuscarinics are used to reduce tremor and rigidity but can worsen tardive dyskinesia. Selegeline has been found to delay the need for levodopa for 9 months but has also been found to increase mortality in another RCT.

22. B **

23. D * This trial was the HOT trial and not CAPRIE trial, which showed that clopidogrel is as effective as aspirin in decreasing the risk of CV events.

24. D ** As sensitivity has 'si' in the word, a useful tip is to associate this with the word sick. As specificity has 'fi' in the word, a useful tip is to associate this with the word fit. The positive predictive value is the proportion of patients with a positive test who have been correctly identified as having the disease.

25. A **

26. C **

27. C *** Guillain-Barré is an example of acute symmetrical peripheral neuropathy, which can be fatal. Patients may not have absent reflexes in the first few hours of the disease. Treatment with intravenous immunoglobulin expedites recovery and reduces disability.

28. B * NNT = 1/ARR% = 1/(% treated group with desired outcome minus % controls with desired outcome). In this example NNT indicates that the increase risk would manifest itself when 20 women are treated.

29. C **

30. A ** Marked elevation of transaminases would have suggested drug hepatotoxicity or viral hepatitis.

31. C **

32. C * The non-steroidal aromatase inhibitors are licensed as alternatives to tamoxifen for the treatment of advanced postmenopausal breast cancer.

33. D *

34. A **

35. D **

36. D **

37. C **

38. C ***

39. E * This is an incidental finding and does not require further investigation or treatment.

40. E **

41. B *

42. C **

43. B * Leflunomide is a new DMD (disease modifying drug) for the treatment of rheumatoid arthritis. It is very popular in the USA and is now available on NHS prescription. The patient's BP and serum LFTs should be monitored.

44. E * Serum IgE is also a valid test.

45. D **

46. C ** Radionuclide bone scans will show this march fracture.

47. E **

48. A *

49. C **

50. E **

51. A *

52. E ***

53. C * Both broccoli and spinach affect INR and patients on warfarin should be advised.

54. A **

55. C ** Structural abnormalities such as MV prolapse and ruptured chordae are now more common than rheumatic heart disease. The murmur is often not the classic pan-systolic, loudest at the apex and radiating into the axilla.

56. B * Endomyocardial biopsies are usually taken from the septal region and therefore may be negative despite RV involvement.

57. C ** Option D is the definition of attributable risk and option E is the definition of absolute risk.

58. D **

59. C *** Pulmonary embolism may be associated with hypotension.

60. B *

61. C **

62. E **

63. B **

64. E *

65. D *** This lady may have primary biliary cirrhosis, a slow, chronic disease.

66. A **

67. A **

68. B * The FSH and LH tests should be performed in the early follicular phase. If >10 IU/L, the patient should receive an early referral to the infertility clinic.

69. B *** This gentleman may have Wegener's granulomatosis.

70. C * For women it is 210 minus the patient's age.

71. B ***

72. E ** If her peak flow does not improve, admit her.

73. B ** According to 'Treating to Target' guidance launched at the Diabetes UK Conference in 2003, a step-up treatment is advised if HbA1C is persistently >7.

74. A ** Topical treatment is suggested for at least 3 months. Alternative topical treatment is zineryt (erythromycin and zinc).

75. A ** The opposite is true.

76. B * Buspirone may improve symptoms in the short term.

77. A * Squamous cell cancer of the head and neck constitutes 5% of all cancers in the UK. People in their forties and fifties are most at risk. Risk factors include alcohol, smoking and having a poor diet.

78. A **

79. C **

80. C *** Tickly cough is a side-effect of ACE inhibitors, in which case an antiotensin-II receptor antagonist may be substituted.

81. B *** Hyperkalaemia and not hypokalaemia is a sign of Addison's disease.

82. B *

83. A *

84. B **

85. B ***

86. D **

87. B *

88. A ***

89. A * Patients with OSA may be treated conservatively with CPAP or offered uvulopalatopharyngoplasty (UPPP) or laser-assisted uvulopalatoplasty (LAUP) if the uvula is redundant with low-hanging soft tissues of the soft palate.

90. D **

91. E ** Hydroxyurea is then prescribed if the platelet count or white cell count is difficult to control.

92. E * The painful arc sign is elicited between 60 and 120 degrees of abduction.

93. D *** Sunlight exposure improves psoriasis.

94. B * Lamellar splitting results from detergents, trauma or water.

95. B *** This man will most likely have an atypical pneumonia. If this infection does not clear, he will require a chest x-ray to exclude tuberculosis.

96. C ** A postmenopausal woman with kyphosis has osteoporosis and does not require a dexa scan to confirm this diagnosis. Weekly alendronate is the preferred treatment for advanced osteoporosis.

97. A * This subungual or periungual topical therapy is applied for 2 months. Mometasone furoate (Elocon) lotion is an alternative.

98. C *** Unilateral wheeze indicates carcinoma of the lung until proven otherwise. This patient may have a normal chest x-ray and still have lung cancer. Bronchoscopy is indicated in a patient with unilateral wheeze.

99. B *** This gentleman most likely has haemochromatosis. The definitive investigation is a liver biopsy. Diabetes mellitus should be excluded.

100. D * Generic prescribing enables any suitable product to be dispensed. Exceptions arise where bioavailability problems occur as in some slow- or modified-release formulations where the patient should always receive the same brand or manfacturer which should therefore be stated in the doctor's prescription.

$\frac{5}{100}$

MRCP Paper Nine BOFs

In these questions candidates must select one answer only

Questions

1. The most effective treatment for Bowen's disease on the lower leg is

   A diclofenac gel
   B fluorouracil cream
   C intradermal triamcinolone
   D self-adhesive silicone gel (Mepiform)
   E tretinoin cream

2. A 55-year-old man has a history of heart failure and requires anti-hypertensive therapy. The single most appropriate antihypertensive drug based on evidence is

   A ACE inhibitor
   B angiotensin-II receptor antagonist
   C beta-blocker
   D calcium antagonist
   E thiazide

3. According to evidence-based treatment of metastatic breast carcinoma, the most appropriate treatment option for relapse on tamoxifen is

   A high-dose chemotherapy
   B paclitaxel
   C radiotherapy
   D standard dose chemotherapy
   E trilostane

4. The following types of dressings may be used for the treatment of chronic wounds (including venous ulcers and pressure sores) EXCEPT

   A alginate
   B hydrocolloid
   C hydrogel
   D polyurethane foam
   E vapour-permeable adhesive

5. The most effective treatment for bullous pemphigoid is

   A dapsone
   B topical fluorouracil (Efudix)
   C hydrocortisone
   D intradermal triamcinolone
   E prednisolone

6. 40 out of 200 heroin misusers in the group treated with buprenor-phine (Subutex) give up heroin and 4 out of 200 give up heroin in the control group. The absolute risk reduction percentage is

   A 5
   B 6
   C 10
   D 18
   E 36

7. 40 out of 200 heroin misusers in the group treated with buprenor-phine (Subutex) give up heroin and 4 out of 200 give up heroin in the control group. The numbers needed to treat (NNT) is

   A 5
   B 6
   C 10
   D 18
   E 36

8. An 80-year-old woman presents with loin pain, haematuria and fever. She was well a month prior. Her ESR is elevated and she has fundoscopic features of giant cell arteritis. Renal biopsy reveals a focal necrotizing GN with crescent formation. The most likely diagnosis is

   A focal segmental glomerulosclerosis
   B mesangiocapillary glomerulonephritis
   C minimal change glomerulonephritis
   D proliferative GN
   E rapidly progressive GN

9. The SINGLE correct statement regarding central retinal vein occlusion is

   A It causes painless loss of vision.
   B It is less common than arterial occlusion.
   C The fundus appears like a stormy red sea.
   D There is no definitive treatment.
   E There is cupping of the optic disc.

10. The following are signs of diabetic retinopathy EXCEPT

    A arteriovenous nipping
    B microaneurysms
    C neovascularisation
    D soft exudates
    E yellow hard exudates

11. Drug levels are required to monitor all of the following medications EXCEPT

    A carbamazepine
    B ciclosporin
    C digoxin
    D lithium
    E theophylline

12. The following statements are correct regarding severe acute respiratory syndrome (SARS) EXCEPT

    A Chest x-ray shows changes suggestive of pneumonia.
    B Early antibiotic intervention is effective.
    C The incubation period is between 2 and 7 days.
    D There have been documented mortalities in Hong Kong and Vietnam.
    E 20 ml of blood in a plain glass tube should be taken.

13. The following blood test is NOT indicated in a patient suspected of having Alzheimer's disease

    A Bone profile
    B FBC + ESR
    C LFTs
    D TFTs
    E U+E + glucose

14. The most effective method for detecting the hepatitis C viral RNA genome is

    A elevated alanine-amino transferase
    B elevated aspartate-amino transferase
    C ELISA-3 blood test
    D liver biopsy
    E polymerase chain reaction (PCR)

15. Causes of monocular diplopia include all of the following EXCEPT

    A astigmatism
    B cataract
    C dislocated lens
    D pterygium
    E strabismus

16. Bisphosphonates are indicated for all of the following conditions EXCEPT

    A inflammatory bowel conditions requiring oral corticosteroids
    B postmenopausal osteoporosis
    C postmenopausal Moslem women
    D premenopausal women with a family history of osteoporosis
    E prolonged oral corticosteroid use for more than 3 months

17. A patient has been recently started on methotrexate for rheumatoid arthritis. He has regular FBC tests. Initial FBC: WCC was 8×10^9/L and platelets 220×10^9/L. Two months later the WCC is 3×10^9/L and the platelets 100×10^9/L. The SINGLE most appropriate management plan is

    A continue current dose of methotrexate
    B decrease by 2.5 mg weekly
    C discontinue methotrexate
    D increase by 2.5 mg weekly
    E none of the above

18. A 70-year-old woman presents with a cloudy cornea, reduced visual acuity and painful red eye. The most likely diagnosis is

    A acute iritis
    B central retinal artery occlusion
    C closed angle glaucoma
    D retinal detachment
    E vitreous haemorrhage

19. A 70-year-old woman presents with swollen lower legs. She is on 5 mg of felodipine for hypertension and indomethacin for rheumatic disease. BP is currently 140/70. The SINGLE most appropriate step is

    A add a loop diuretic
    B add a thiazide diuretic
    C change felodipine to an ACE inhibitor
    D change indometacin to a Cox 2 inhibitor
    E prescribe elastic stockings

20. A 22-year-old man has persistent otitis externa. He enjoys swimming. He has been using dexamethasone and neomycin spray (Otomize). The ear swab reveals pseudomonas aeruginosa. The SINGLE best management option is

A add amoxicillin
B add ciprofloxacin
C add trimethoprim
D advise him to wear ear plugs when swimming
E change to dexamethasone and framycetin and gramicidin otic drops (Sofradex)

21. A 20-year-old professional rugby player develops infectious mononucleosis. He wants to know when it will be safe to go back to contact sports. The SINGLE best management option is

A advise to wait 6 weeks
B advise to wait 3 months
C advise to return when monospot test is negative
D arrange for an ultrasound of the spleen to exclude splenomegaly
E arrange for a CT scan of the liver and spleen

22. The following are appropriate diagnostic investigations for fever following tropical travel EXCEPT

A CRP
B three EDTA samples to haematology for thick and thin films
C malaria serology
D stool for parasites and culture with mention of countries visited
E tropical serology for schistosomiasis

23. The following statements on statistics are correct EXCEPT

A A case referent study looks back from disease to exposure and gives a comparison of incidence rates.
B A cohort study looks forward from exposure to disease.
C Both relative risk and odds ratio can be determined using a cross-sectional study.
D The incidence rate is defined as the number of new cases in a given period divided by the total person time at risk during the period.
E The odds ratio is good for studying large populations and rare diseases.

24. A 16-year-old girl presents with persistent productive cough for 4 months with no relief from repeated courses of antibiotics. On chest examination she has occasional wheezes. The following investigations should be arranged EXCEPT

A chest x-ray
B peak flow meter
C spirometry
D sweat test
E salbutamol therapeutic trial

25. Prophylactic antibiotics should be prescribed in HIV+ patients if the CD4 count drops below

A 100 cells/mm^3
B 200 cells/mm^3
C 300 cells/mm^3
D 400 cells/mm^3
E 500 cells/mm^3

26. The following statements regarding ECG arrhythmias are correct EXCEPT

A In atrial flutter, the atrial rate is between 350 and 600 beats/min and the ventricular rate is between 100 and 180 beats/min.
B In atrial fibrillation, the P waves are absent.
C In Wolff–Parkinson–White syndrome, the atrial impulses can be conducted via the accessory pathway, causing ventricular pre-excitation and broad QRS complexes with delta waves.
D In Wolff–Parkinson–White syndrome, the patient is at risk of ventricular fibrillation.
E Ventricular tachycardia is defined as three or more ventricular extrasystoles in succession at a rate of more than 120 beats/min.

27. A 56-year-old obese man presents with sudden onset of severe back pain. He has no signs of sciatica or urinary incontinence. BP is 150/90. Possible diagnoses include all of the following EXCEPT

A acute pancreatitis
B cord compression
C renal colic
D ruptured abdominal aortic aneurysm
E simple mechanical back pain

28. A 14-year-old girl presents with severe acne over her face, arms and back. She has tried 3 months of topical therapy without success. The most appropriate treatment in addition to co-cyprindiol (Dianette) and adapalene (Differin) would be

A oral erythromycin (Erythroped)
B oxytetracycline
C isotretinoin (Roaccutane)
D trimethoprim
E topical erythromycin (Zineryt)

29. Select the SINGLE most appropriate interpretation for the following HBV serology result

    sAb +ve   sAg –ve   cAb –ve   eAg –ve   eAb –ve   DNA –ve

A immune, post-vaccination
B immune, past exposure to HBV
C infected, low risk of transmission
D infected, high risk of transmission
E none of the above

30. A 60-year-old woman is seen in rheumatology clinic. She has a past history of hip fracture. You decide to put her on medication for osteoporosis. Besides calcichew D3 forte, you should add

A alendronic acid
B calcitonin
C hormone replacement therapy (HRT)
D raloxifine
E tiludronic acid

31. A 40-year-old woman reports facial flushing. On examination she has erythema, papules, pustules and telangiectasia on the nose and cheeks. The facial flushing is made worse by alcohol and sun exposure. The most likely diagnosis is

A acne vulgaris
B sarcoidosis
C discoid lupus erythematosus
D psoriasis
E rosacea

32. A 35-year-old woman with no alarm symptoms presents with 4 weeks of dyspepsia despite antacid therapy. The most appropriate investigation is

    A double-contrast barium meal (DCBM)
    B endoscopy
    C gastric parietal cell antibody
    D *Helicobacter pylori* serology
    E urea breath test

33. Alarm symptoms as to the cause of dyspepsia include all of the following EXCEPT

    A Barrett's oesophagus
    B 45-year-old with positive *Helicobacter pylori* test
    C dysphagia
    D jaundice
    E peptic ulcer surgery >20 years ago

34. The SINGLE best drug for treatment for social phobia is

    A diazepam
    B fluoxetine
    C moclobemide
    D paroxetine
    E phenelzine

35. All the following conditions may be associated with alopecia EXCEPT

    A chronic iron deficiency
    B fungal scalp infection
    C hyperthyroidism
    D polycystic ovarian syndrome
    E warfarin

36. The following statements regarding the management of breast cancer are correct EXCEPT

    A A positive sentinel node biopsy for locoregional breast cancer requires axillary node clearance and no radiotherapy.
    B Locoregional breast cancer can be treated by wide local excision or mastectomy + radiotherapy.
    C Node-negative systemic breast cancer in a premenopausal female should be offered chemotherapy.
    D Node-positive systemic breast cancer requires chemotherapy ± zoladex in a premenopausal female.
    E Node-positive systemic breast cancer in a postmenopausal female should be offered tamoxifen ± chemotherapy.

37. A 60-year-old man presents with jaundice, pale stools and dark urine following laparoscopic cholecystectomy. Ultrasound reveals dilated common bile duct. The SINGLE most discrimating investigation is

A ERCP
B liver biopsy
C blood cultures
D percutaneous transhepatic cholangiography
E viral serology

38. The following are risk factors for a patient's risk of being a danger to others EXCEPT

A evidence of general self-neglect
B lack of remorse regarding violence
C morbid jealousy
D past history of violence with alcohol or drugs
E persisting denial of responsibility

39. The following statements regarding buprenorphine (Subutex) are correct EXCEPT

A It is a Class C drug according to the Misuse of Drugs Act 1971.
B It may be used as substitution therapy for patients with moderate opioid dependence.
C It should initially be administered in hospital.
D Patients on methadone should be down to 30 mg of methadone od prior to conversion to buprenorphine
E It should be taken at least 4 hours after last use of opioid.

40. A 30-year-old woman presents with three recurrent miscarriages. She also suffers from chronic migraines. The investigation that is most likely to lead to the underlying diagnosis is

A anti-mitochondrial antibody
B anti-neutrophil cytoplasmic antibody
C anti-nuclear antibody
D anti-phospholipid antibody
E antibody to reticulin

41. The following are causes of hypercalcaemia EXCEPT

A bone metastases
B Conn's syndrome
C primary hyperparathyroidism
D sarcoidosis
E thyrotoxicosis

42. The following tests are useful for the investigation of hypercalcaemia EXCEPT

    A full blood count
    B isotope bone scan
    C chest x-ray
    D 12-lead ECG
    E thyroid function tests

43. The initial investigation for polyuria (>3 L/day) should be

    A fasting blood glucose
    B MSU for culture and sensitivities
    C serum calcium
    D urea and electrolytes
    E urine dipstick

44. The following may suggest thyroid malignancy EXCEPT

    A family history of thyroid cancer
    B hoarseness>6 weeks
    C cervical lymphadenopathy
    D overt thyroid dysfunction
    E prior irradiation to the neck

45. The following conditions are associated with erectile dysfunction EXCEPT

    A adrenal insufficiency
    B Cushing's syndrome
    C diabetes mellitus
    D hyperprolactinaemia
    E phaeochromocytoma

46. A 50-year-old obese woman is noted to have persistent hypertension. You suspect Cushing's, as she has abdominal striae. The single routine biochemical blood test result which would most support the diagnosis is

    A hypercholesterolaemia
    B hyperglycaemia
    C hypocalcaemia
    D hyponatraemia
    E hypokalaemia

47. The SINGLE best treatment for acute cluster headache is

    A paracetamol
    B ergotamine
    C lithium carbonate
    D methysergide
    E sumatriptan

48. The definitive test in the investigation of repeat haemoptysis is

    A bronchoscopy
    B chest x-ray
    C chest CT scan
    D sputum for AFB (acid-fast bacilli)
    E sputum for C+S

49. Of the following the most worrying sign that a mole may be a melanoma is

    A bleeding mole
    B change in shape
    C diameter >7 mm
    D more than one shade of pigment present
    E sensory change

50. Carpal tunnel syndrome is associated with all of the following conditions EXCEPT

    A acromegaly
    B amyloidosis
    C hypothyroidism
    D multiple sclerosis
    E rheumatoid arthritis

51. The following statements regarding liver tumours are correct EXCEPT

    A Alcohol injection into the tumour may be used as an interim measure prior to liver transplantation.
    B Anti-retroviral therapy is required post-liver transplant.
    C In the UK, 75% of hepatocellular carcinoma is associated with hepatitis C.
    D Large tumours recur quickly even after liver transplantation.
    E Radiofrequency ablation is the best treatment for small liver tumours.

52. Risk factors for gallstones include all of the following EXCEPT

    A diabetes mellitus
    B haemolytic disease
    C obesity
    D peptic ulcer disease
    E type IV hyperlipidaemia

53. The following statements regarding pancreatic cancer are correct EXCEPT

    A A high serum CA-19.9 is highly suggestive of pancreatic cancer.
    B Chemotherapy has a limited effect on survival rates.
    C Cancers in the body of the pancreas are often resectable.
    D The most common presentation is obstructive jaundice.
    E The most common site is the head of the pancreas.

54. A 55-year-old man on bendrofluazide for hypertension now presents with cough, orthopnoea and paroxysmal nocturnal dyspnoea. Chest examination reveals basal rales. The single most appropriate treatment option is

    A furosemide (frusemide)
    B losartan
    C prednisolone
    D ramipril
    E spironolactone

55. The most common cause of cellulitis in adults is infection with

    A *Haemophilus influenzae*
    B *Pseudomonas aeruginosa*
    C *Staphlylococcus aureus*
    D *Staphylococcus epidermidis*
    E *Streptococcus pyogenes*

56. The most appropriate treatment for erysipelas is

    A ampicillin
    B ciprofloxacin
    C erythromycin
    D flucloxacillin
    E phenoxymethylpenicillin

57. The following statements regarding multiple sclerosis are correct EXCEPT

   A CSF electrophoresis reveals the presence of oligoclonal bands.
   B It is due to the demyelination of the peripheral nervous system.
   C It often presents with a rapid deterioration of central vision.
   D MRI scan of the brain is diagnostic.
   E Interferon beta-1b and glatiramer acetate reduce relapse by 30% and reduce the rate of the appearance of new lesions.

58. Acute management of cluster headaches involves oxygen 100% at 7 L/min and

   A analgaesia
   B ergotamine
   C prednisolone
   D sumatriptan
   E verapamil

59. Recognised prophylactic drugs for migraine include all of the following EXCEPT

   A amitriptyline
   B beta-blockers
   C mefenamic acid
   D sodium valproate
   E pizotifen

60. The SINGLE most effective treatment for candida paronychia is

   A calcipotriol (Dovonex) scalp solution
   B gloves and moisturiser
   C terbinafine (Lamisil)
   D itraconazole (Sporonox)
   E topical steroid

61. The following statements regarding heart failure are correct EXCEPT

    A All patients with heart failure due to LV systolic dysfunction should be considered for treatment with an ACE inhibitor.

    B Beta-blockers licensed for use in heart failure should be initiated in patients with heart failure due to LV systolic dysfunction after diuretic and ACE inhibitor therapy, regardless of whether symptoms persist or not.

    C Diagnosis should be confirmed by Doppler 2D echocardiographic examination to exclude valve disease, assess LV function and detect intracardiac shunts.

    D Patients with heart failure due to diastolic dysfunction should usually be treated with a loop diuretic.

    E Patients with heart failure should be offered annual pneumococcal vaccination.

62. A 20-year-old male presents with photophobia and red eye after a blunt blow to the right eye socket. On examination there is a hyphaema in the anterior uvea. He is at high risk of

    A increased intraocular pressure
    B optic nerve damage
    C orbital blowout fracture
    D orbital abscess
    E papilloedema

63. A 22-year-old male presents with red eye, irregular pupil and photophobia. On examination he is noted to have panuveitis. The investigation that would be most helpful in reaching a diagnosis is

    A anti-nuclear antibody
    B ESR
    C full blood count
    D HLA B27
    E rheumatoid factor

64. The most effective form of treatment for plaque psoriasis is

    A coal tar preparation
    B dithranol
    C vitamin D analogue/corticosteroid (Dovobet)
    D calcipotriol (Dovonex)
    E emollient

65. Psoriasis may be associated with all of the following EXCEPT

   A anterior uveitis
   B fungal nail infection
   C geographical tongue
   D joint arthropathy
   E pustules on the palms

66. A 20-year-old woman presents with a rash following a streptococcal throat infection. She has completed a week's course of amoxicillin. On examination there are multiple 1-cm-round raised red patches over her abdomen. The most likely diagnosis is

   A dermatophytosis
   B erythema multiforme
   C guttate psoriasis
   D infectious mononucleosis
   E pityriasis rosea

67. A 55-year-old brick layer presents with a superficial nodule over his right upper eyelid. On examination there is also absence of eyelashes underlying the nodule. This lesion is most suspicious of

   A basal cell carcinoma
   B chalazion cyst
   C melanoma
   D solitary plaque of psoriasis
   E squamous cell carcinoma

68. A 60-year-old South Asian female presents with fatigue and short-ness of breath. Full blood count reveals a Hb 11 g/dl, MCV 70 fl and a MCHC 28 g/dl. Further investigations should include all of the fol-lowing EXCEPT

   A blood film
   B checking for faecal occult blood
   C serum ferritin
   D serum total iron binding capacity
   E urine dipstick testing

69. The following statements regarding metoclopramide are correct EXCEPT

   A Domperidone is unlikely to work if metoclopramide fails.
   B It is useful for gastric stasis.
   C It should be avoided in mechanical bowel obstruction.
   D Metoclopramide and cyclizine may be taken together.
   E Side-effects are counteracted by procyclidine.

70. The following are risk factors for osteoporosis EXCEPT

   A inflammatory bowel disease
   B maternal hip fracture
   C natural menopause before age 45 years
   D psoriasis
   E rheumatoid arthritis

71. The following statements regarding the management of osteoporosis are correct EXCEPT

   A Bisphosphonates act by blocking osteoclast action.
   B Calcitonin is an endogenous inhibitor of bone resorption.
   C Salmon calcitonin is available as a nasal spray.
   D Salmon calcitonin is 10 times more potent than normally produced human calcitonin.
   E Selective oestrogen receptor modulators have been shown to decrease non-vertebral fractures in postmenopausal women.

72. According to the British Society of Gastroenterology, the following statements regarding the management of dyspepsia are correct EXCEPT

   A Patients under the age of 55 with uncomplicated dyspepsia on the basis of a positive *H. pylori* test do not require endoscopy prior to treatment.
   B The ^{13}C urea breath test must not be performed within 4 weeks of antibiotic use.
   C The most accurate test for identification of and for confirmation of eradication of *H. pylori* is the serological test demonstrating antibodies to the organism.
   D The national cancer referral guidance recommends endoscopy for new dyspepsia in patients over the age of 55.
   E Treatment should be stopped 4 weeks before endoscopy.

73. The most common diagnosis made at endoscopy for dyspepsia in all age groups is

   A duodenal or gastric ulcer
   B gastritis or duodenitis
   C hiatal hernia
   D oesophagitis
   E normal

74. A 20-year-old man presents with swinging fever, non-productive cough and tender subcutaneous nodules on his shins. Chest x-ray shows bilateral hilar lymphodenopathy. The MOST appropriate treatment is

A amoxicillin
B clarithromycin
C co-fluampicil
D prednisolone
E rifampicin, isoniazid and pyrazinamide

75. Clinical signs of alcoholic liver disease include all of the following EXCEPT

A Dupuytren's contracture
B palmar erythema
C parotid enlargement
D erythropoietic protoporphyria
E spider naevi

76. Potential side-effects of amiodarone include all of the following EXCEPT

A agranulocytosis
B fatty liver
C optic neuritis
D pneumonitis
E thyroid dysfunction

77. Risk factors for gastric cancer include all of the following EXCEPT

A asbestos exposure
B achalasia
C blood group A
D pernicious anaemia
E smoked foods

78. The following investigations may be used to stage gastric cancer EXCEPT

A CT scan of abdomen
B double contrast barium meal
C endoscopic ultrasound
D laparoscopy with laparoscopic ultrasound
E PET (positive emission tomography scanning)

79. The following statements regarding allergic rhinitis are correct EXCEPT

    A H1-antihistamines are recommended as first-line treatment.
    B It is a type I hypersensitivity reaction to aeroallergen.
    C Leukotriene receptor antagonists (LTRAs) may be offered to those who fail to respond to topical corticosteroids and H1-antihistamines.
    D In children, intranasal fluticasone suppresses the hypothalamic–pituitary axis.
    E The most common allergen in perennial allergic rhinitis in the UK is grass pollen.

80. Rheumatoid arthritis may be associated with all of the following EXCEPT

    A atlanto-axial instability
    B iritis
    C morning joint stiffness
    D pleural effusion
    E septic arthritis

81. Trigger finger may be associated with all of the following conditions EXCEPT

    A carpal tunnel syndrome
    B diabetes mellitus
    C haemodialysis
    D lederhosen syndrome
    E rheumatoid arthritis

82. Conditions associated with Dupuytren's contracture include all of the following EXCEPT

    A amyloidosis
    B diabetes mellitus
    C epilepsy
    D HIV infection
    E Peyronie's disease

83. Polycystic ovary syndrome is associated with an increase in values of all of the following blood tests EXCEPT

    A free testosterone
    B LH/FSH ratio
    C luteinising hormone
    D oestrone–oestradiol ratio
    E sex hormone binding globulins

84. A 45-year-old woman reports pain radiating down the anterolateral side of her right thigh with decreased sensitivity to touch. The pain is aggravated by walking and relieved by lying down with the hip flexed. On examination motor function is normal. The most likely diagnosis is

A malingering
B meralgia paraesthetica
C multiple sclerosis
D osteoarthritis of the hip
E sciatica

85. Diagnostic criteria for polymyalgia rheumatica include all of the following EXCEPT

A age below 60 years
B morning stiffness lasting more than an hour
C pain persisting for more than 1 month involving two areas of the neck, shoulders and pelvic girdle
D prompt response to prednisolone (<20 mg/day)
E Westergreen ESR >40 mm/h

86. A 35-year-old woman with SLE presents with renal impairment. Renal biopsy reveals thickened basement membrane, IF +ve for IgG and C3 and subepithelial deposits on EM. The most likely diagnosis is

A focal segmental glomerulosclerosis
B mesangiocapillary glomerulonephritis
C membranous nephropathy
D minimal change glomerulonephritis
E rapidly progressive glomerulonephritis

87. The following are cardinal signs of glaucoma EXCEPT

A increased intraocular pressure
B optic disc cupping
C eye pain
D squint
E visual field constriction

88. The following statements regarding the management of Alzheimer's disease (AD) are correct EXCEPT

   A Apolipoprotein e4 allele is associated with an increased likelihood of developing AD.
   B Measurement of medial temporal lobe thickness on temporal lobe-oriented scans allows definitive diagnosis.
   C Memantine is a non-competitive NMDA (glutamate) receptor antagonist used for severe AD.
   D Rivastigmine may be offered for management of mild and moderate AD.
   E There is characteristic asymmetrical bilateral temporo-parietal hypoperfusion on SPECT (single photon emission computed tomography).

89. The following drugs may be used in prophylaxis against malaria EXCEPT

   A chloroquine + proguanil hydrochloride
   B doxycycline
   C mefloquine (Lariam)
   D proquanil with atovaquone (malarone)
   E quinine

90. Potential complications of malaria include all of the following complications EXCEPT

   A cirrhosis
   B hypoglycaemia
   C nephrotic syndrome
   D pulmonary oedema
   E splenic rupture

91. 1000 individuals were observed for a period of 20 years. 150 out of the 200 who worked in a shipyard developed mesothelioma; 8 of the 800 who did not work in a shipyard went on to develop mesothelioma. The risk ratio is

   A 7.5
   B 15
   C 37.5
   D 75
   E 150

92. The following statements are correct regarding odds ratio EXCEPT

   A It can be calculated from a cohort study.
   B It is good for large populations.
   C It is good for rare diseases.
   D It is defined as the number of new cases in a given period divided by the total persons with disease during a given period.
   E It needs a control group.

93. The following conditions require adrenaline (epinephrine) administration in the management of anaphylaxis EXCEPT

   A bronchospasm
   B facial angio-oedema
   C hypotension
   D laryngeal oedema
   E shock

94. The following drugs should be considered in the medical treatment of peripheral arterial disease EXCEPT

   A ACE inhibitors
   B clopidogrel
   C beta-blocker
   D cilostazol
   E statin

95. A 60-year-old woman is noted to have iron-deficiency anaemia. Upper gastro intestinal (UGI) endoscopy and barium enema are both normal. The next investigation should be

   A CT scan of abdomen
   B colonoscopy
   C proctoscopy
   D sigmoidoscopy
   E ultrasound of abdomen

96. Notifiable diseases include all of the following EXCEPT

   A anthrax
   B Lyme disease
   C measles
   D meningitis
   E tuberculosis

97. A 20-year-old man complains of pain following a treated animal bite to the leg. Symptoms are characterised by spontaneous pain with hyperalgesia, abnormal sweating, loss of function, oedema and skin blood flow abnormalities. On examination there is no injury to a major nerve. The most likely diagnosis is

A complex regional pain syndrome (reflex sympathetic dystrophy)
B deafferentation pain
C fibromyalgia
D incidental post-herpetic neuralgia
E psychological pain syndrome

98. Polycythaemia rubra vera is associated with an increase in all of the following tests EXCEPT

A serum vitamin B_{12}
B leucocyte alkaline phosphatose (LAP)
C platelets
D plasma volume
E red cell mass

99. A 60-year-old man attends A+E with abrupt onset of severe left-sided flank pain. He has a past history of renal colic. He is afebrile. AXR is negative. The urine dipstick is positive for blood and white cells. The analgaesia of choice is

A cocodamol PO
B diclofenac IM
C morphine PR
D pethidine IM
E tramadol PO

100. A 30-year-old man presents with six month persistent unproductive nocturnal cough. His FEV_1 is 70% of predicted but chest examination and x-ray are normal. The most appropriate treatment is

A amoxicillin
B clarithromycin
C ipratropium inhaler
D prednisolone
E salbutamol inhaler

Answers to BOFs Paper Nine

Criterion Referencing Marks

    *   – 25–50% of candidates expected to get correct
    **   – 50–75% of candidates expected to get correct
    *** – 75–100% of candidates expected to get correct

The notional PASS MARK is 62%

---

1. B * Excision and grafting is an alternative treatment.

2. A ***

3. B * Paclitaxel is a taxane and is the treatment of choice for ovarian cancer. Both paclitaxel and docetaxel are also used for the treatment of advanced or metastatic breast cancer as per NICE guidelines. Trilostane has a minor role in post-menopausal breast cancer that has relapsed following oestrogen antagonist therapy. As it inhibits the synthesis of glucocorticoids and mineralocorticoids, concomitant cortiscosteroid replacement therapy is required.

4. E *

5. E ** Azathioprine may also be added.

6. D ** 20% – 2% = 18%

7. B * 1/18% = 5.56 or 6 people

8. E ** Treatment involves high-dose corticosteroids, cyclophosphamide ± plasma exchange or renal transplant. Prognosis is poor if the initial serum creatinine level is >600 µmol/1.

9. C ** Visual acuity may be reduced to finger counting.

10. A ** Degrees of diabetic retinopathy increase in severity from BDR (background retinopathy distinguished by the presence of microaneurysms), preproliferative retinopathy (presence of lipoproteins as hard exudates, soft exudates) to proliferative retinopathy with neovascularisation. As new vessels are at risk of bleeding, i.e. vitreous haemorrhage or forming scar tissue, and may result in permanent vision loss, diabetic patients should be followed closely with annual specialist eye examinations. Laser treatment is used to get closure of leaky blood vessels or microaneurysms. Panretinal photocoagulation is used to treat neovascularisation.

11. A **

12. B ** Blood should be taken during the acute and convalescent phase (14 days later) with a 20-ml sample of urine and sent to the lab marked suspected SARS. There is no cure or prophylactic treatment as yet. SARS is a notifiable disease of exclusion.

13. A ***

14. D ** In October 2003, NICE reviewed combination treatment of once-weekly pegylated interferon. Currently the only licensed treatment of hepatitis C is interferon alfa. Combination therapy involves oral ribavarin in combination with interferon alfa 2a or 2b.

15. E **

16. D * Once-weekly alendronate (Fosamax) is a convenient form of bisphosphonate therapy. Exercise should be advocated in premenopausal women.

17. C ** Medication errors have occurred with methotrexate. Note it is a once-weekly drug! Methotrexate must be stopped if any profound drop in WCC or platelets occurs.

18. A **

19. D **

20. B **

21. D *

22. C *** Malaria serology is unhelpful as a diagnostic aid and is very rarely indicated. Initial investigation should always be three EDTA tubes for blood film. 1% of cases are now due to HIV seroconversion, which will show atypical lymphocytes on film. Suspect if the patient has a rash.

23. C * Both relative risk and odds ratio can be determined with a cohort study. However this is time consuming.

24. D ***

25. B ** These patients will be at risk of developing pneumocystis carinii pneumonia and co-trimoxazole should be prescribed.

26. A ** This describes atrial fibrillation not flutter.

27. B ** Beware sudden onset of severe back pain in men over the age of 55. Do not forget to examine the abdomen for a pulsatile aneurysm.

28. A ** Trimethoprim is reserved for antibiotic-resistant acne. Triple therapy is advised for 3 months, at which time the erythromycin should be reduced to once daily for 1 month and then discontinued. Adapalene (Differin) gel should be applied thinly and continued as prophylaxis.

29. A **

30. A * Alendronic acid and risedronate (both bisphosphonates) are available as once-weekly preparations, which is more amenable for patients who dislike daily tablets. The classic Dowager's hump is pathognomonic for severe osteoporosis without imaging. A lateral back x-ray should be obtained if osteoporosis is suspected and confirmed by dexa scan. A value ≥ 2.5 standard deviations below the young adult female value is the WHO definition for osteoporosis. It is deemed negligence if you do not put your patient on osteoporosis prophylaxis if you prescribe long-term corticosteroids. Recent evidence shows that repeated short courses of steroids may be more detrimental than long-term regular steroids! HRT is no longer recommended as prophylaxis against osteoporosis and should only be prescribed 2–3 years maximum, for relief of troublesome menopausal symptoms.

31. E **

32. E **

33. B *** Guidelines for endoscopy have now changed to age 55.

34. D * Moclobemide, a reversible MAOI, should be reserved for second-line treatment.

35. C ** Hypothyroidism leads to poor hair growth and a coarsening of the hair shaft. The most common cause is fungal scalp infections.

36. C * For this patient, treatment option may or may not involve chemotherapy.

37. A *** This gentleman most likely has a stone in the common bile duct.

38. A *** This is a risk factor for self-harm.

39. C ** It may be prescribed in an outpatient clinic. It is advisable that the patient should also be involved with a community drug team.

40. C ***

41. B *** Conn's syndrome is associated with hyperaldosteronism.

42. D *** Serum urea and electrolytes and liver function tests should also be obtained.

43. A ***

44. D ** Overt thyroid dysfunction lessens the risk of malignancy.

45. E *

46. E ***

47. E * The rest are examples of prophylactic treatment except for analgaesia, which plays no role in the treatment of cluster headaches.

48. A ***

49. B * The UK major signs of melanoma are changes to size, shape and colour. The other signs are minor signs. One major sign or three or four minor signs are required for urgent referral to dermatology.

50. D ***

51. E * This is still under investigation as an alternative to surgery.

52. D ***

53. C ** Tumour in the body of the pancreas usually presents with advanced inoperable disease.

54. D *** This gentleman is presenting with signs of heart failure and would benefit from an ACE inhibitor.

55. E **

56. E **

57. B *** MS is a disease of demyelination of the central nervous system.

58. D * 6 mg of sumatriptan SC is advocated for acute treatment of cluster headaches. Analgaesia is not recommended!

59. C *** Mefenamic acid is used for menstrually related migraine.

60. D * Itraconazole is prescribed as 200 mg bd 7/7, repeat monthly for 2 pulses.

61. E * Patients with heart failure should receive annual vaccination against influenza but only a one-off vaccination against pneumococcus. This is based on the NICE guidelines for the management of chronic heart failure, July 2003.

62. A * This patient should be seen by an ophthalmologist urgently who may prescribe timolol, atropine and dexamethasone eye drops (Maxidex) if the IOP is raised. The hyphaema represents red blood cells.

63. D **

64. C *

65. B *** Psoriasis is associated with nail pitting and onycholysis but not fungal nail infections.

66. C **

67. A **

68. A **

69. D * Metoclopramide and cyclizine counteract each other.

70. D *** Psoriasis is not a risk factor in itself, unless the patient is on long-term steroid treatment.

71. E ** Raloxifene has been shown to reduce vertebral fracture by 30% in postmenopausal women.

72. C ** ^{13}C urea breath test is the best test to confirm eradication of *H. pylori*.

73. E *** 30% of endoscopies are normal. 30% are a mix of either gastritis, duodenitis or hiatal hernia.

74. D *** This man may have sarcoidosis.

75. D * Porphyria cutanea tarda (PCT) may be inherited (autosomal dominant) or acquired and associated with cirrhosis. Episodes can be precipitated by alcholol, iron overload, oestrogens and hepatitis C. Whereas the defect in porphyrin metabolism is in the liver in PCT, it lies in the bone marrow in erythropoietic protoporphyria though there may be hepatic dysfunction.

76. A *

77. B ** Achalasia is a risk factor for oesophageal carcinoma.

78. B ** Double-contrast barium meal and upper GI endoscopy with brush biopsies and cytology are diagnostic tests and not used for staging.

79. E * House dust mites are most responsible for perennial allergic rhinitis.

80. E **

81. D * This is associated with Dupuytren's contracture and not trigger finger.

82. A * Amyloidosis may be associated with trigger finger.

83. E * SHBG is reduced in this condition.

84. B ** This is due to compression of the lateral cutaneous nerve of the thigh. Steroid injections are effective.

85. A ** Age can be 50 years or older for the diagnosis of PMR to be made.

86. C * Other associations include malignancy, drugs, autoimmune conditions and infections. Treatment involves corticosteroids and chlorambucil (Ponticelli regimen).

87. D ***

88. B * Definitive diagnosis of AD can only be made by neuropathology (presence of neurofibrillary tangles and amyloid plaques).

89. E ** Pyrimethamine with sulfadoxine (Fansidar) and quinine cannot be used for prophylaxis but rather for treatment.

90. A **

91. D ***

92. D ***

93. B * Injudicious use of adrenaline (epinephrine) can precipitate ventricular tachycardia.

94. C *** According to the HOPE (heart outcomes prevention evaluation) study, ramipril, an ACE inhibitor, is very beneficial in peripheral arterial disease.

95. B ***

96. B ***

97. A *

98. D ** Plasma volume is decreased.

99. B ** Although an opiate-based analgaesia + antiemetic IM is also an option.

100. E *** This man would benefit from a trial of salbutamol as he may have nocturnal asthma.

MRCP Paper Ten BOFs

In these questions candidates must select one answer only

Questions

1. Immediate effects following spinal hemisection include all of the following EXCEPT

   A contralateral flaccid paralysis
   B impairment of ipsilateral proprioceptive perception
   C ipsilateral spastic paralysis
   D loss of contralateral touch sensation
   E spinal shock

2. Which one of the following statements regarding surface anatomy is INCORRECT

   A The bifurcation of the aorta is just below the umbilicus.
   B The left lobe of the liver extends into the 5th intercostal space.
   C The middle meningeal artery is located behind the pterion.
   D The neck of the pancreas is at the tip of the 9th costal cartilage.
   E The spleen is normally palpable.

3. The following statements regarding erythropoietin are correct EXCEPT

   A It is metabolised in the liver.
   B It is raised by living at high altitude.
   C It may be raised in cerebellar haemangioma.
   D It is synthesised in the liver.
   E Production is raised in secondary polycythaemia.

4. Autosomal dominant inherited conditions include all of the following EXCEPT

   A achondroplasia
   B dystrophia myotonica
   C Huntington's chorea
   D idiopathic haemochromatosis
   E osteogenesis imperfecta

5. Hepatitis B may be associated with which ONE of the following?

   A an incubation period of up to 12 months
   B carrier status co-infection if HbsAg is present for >3 months
   C Hepatitis D
   D infection with an RNA virus
   E low infectivity if HbeAg is present

6. Insects are vectors which are responsible for all of the following diseases EXCEPT

   A leishmaniasis
   B Lyme disease (*Borrelia burgdorferi*)
   C trypanosomiasis (sleeping sickness)
   D Weil's disease (*Leptospirosis icterohaemorrhagica*)
   E yellow fever

7. Of the following drugs the one which is used in the treatment of HIV infection, and which is a non-nucleoside reverse transcriptase inhibitor, is

   A abacavir
   B nelfinavir
   C nevirapine
   D zidovudine
   E ritonavir

8. The condition which is a cutaneous manifestation of malignancy is

   A dermatitis herpetiformis
   B erythema multiforme
   C necrobiosis lipoidica
   D pemphigoid
   E thrombophlebitis migrans

9. Aims in the management of diabetes mellitus include all of the following EXCEPT

   A a cholesterol level of <2.5 in the elderly
   B a systolic BP of <140 in the elderly
   C an albumin creatinine ratio (ACR) of <3.5 in a female and <2.5 in a male
   D an annual check of HbA1C
   E an explanation that one cigarette for a diabetic is the equivalent of three cigarettes in a non-diabetic

10. Treatment of psoriasis includes all of the following agents EXCEPT

A ciclosporin
B emollients
C topical fluorouracil (Efudix)
D topical steroids
E vitamin D analogue cream

11. Porphyria cutanea tarda is associated with all of the following EXCEPT

A a decrease in activity of hepatic uroporphyrinogen decarboxylase
B haemochromatosis
C linear skin eruptions
D overproduction of uroporphyrins
E trigger factors including alcohol, oestrogens and hepatitis C

12. Agents that cause phytophotodermatitis include all of the following EXCEPT

A celery
B cow parsley
C giant hogweed
D parsnip
E poison ivy

13. The following statements regarding malignant melanoma are correct EXCEPT

A It has a better prognosis if the growth phase is radial as opposed to vertical.
B It has a worse prognosis if it occurs on the back.
C It is treated by block dissection.
D It may be treated with high-dose interferon.
E Staging is by sentinel node biopsy.

14. Pernicious anaemia is characterised by all of the following EXCEPT

A bone marrow hypoplasia
B hyperbilirubinaemia
C hypergastrinaemia
D hypersegmented neutophilia
E pancytopenia

15. All of the following are causes of diffuse pulmonary fibrosis EXCEPT

    A ciclosporin
    B haemosiderosis
    C systemic sclerosis
    D tuberculosis
    E Wegener's granulomatosis

16. Aortic stenosis may be associated with which ONE of the following signs?

    A atrial fibrillation
    B basal diastolic murmur
    C left parasternal heave
    D left ventricular hypertrophy
    E pulmonary hypertension

17. Features of osteitis deformans (Paget's disease) include all of the following EXCEPT

    A deafness
    B increase in hydroxyproline in the urine
    C low calcium and phosphate levels in the serum
    D osteoporosis circumscripta
    E sarcomatous changes

18. Causes of sudden painless loss of vision include all of the following EXCEPT

    A central retinal vein thrombosis
    B giant cell arteritis
    C malignant hypertension
    D retinitis pigmentosa
    E vitreous haemorrhage

19. Acute renal failure is associated with which one of the following findings?

    A hypernatraemia
    B hypokalaemia
    C hypocalcaemia
    D increased urinary sodium excretion
    E polycythaemia

20. Features associated with a meningomyelocele include all of the following EXCEPT

   A congenital dislocation of the hips
   B congenital heart disease
   C hydrocephalus
   D paraplegia
   E pepperpot skull

21. Signs of cerebellopontine angle tumours include all of the following EXCEPT

   A ataxia
   B reduced corneal reflex
   C tinnitus
   D unilateral sensorineural hearing loss
   E visual field defect

22. Multi-infarct dementia is associated with all of the following EXCEPT

   A a familial tendency
   B depersonalisation
   C disorientation to time and place
   D impaired concentration
   E impaired memory retention

23. The following statements regarding retinal detachment are correct EXCEPT

   A It can occur due to melanoma.
   B It is a hazard of the sport of bungee jumping.
   C It is less common in myopic eyes.
   D It may present with field defects.
   E It may present with sudden visual flashes of light.

24. Causes of lung abscess include all of the following EXCEPT

   A achalasia
   B acute osteomyelitis
   C alcoholism
   D mycoplasma pneumonia
   E staphylococcal pneumonia

25. Peripheral neuropathy is associated with all of the following conditions EXCEPT

    A bronchial carcinoma
    B chronic renal failure
    C hyperthyroidism
    D rheumatoid arthritis
    E vitamin B₁ deficiency

26. Neurological causes of dysphagia include all of the following EXCEPT

    A Friedreich's ataxia
    B bulbar palsy
    C lateral medullary syndrome
    D myasthenia gravis
    E syringomyelia

27. The cause of lateral medullary syndrome is due to the occlusion of

    A anterior cerebral artery
    B internal carotid artery
    C middle cerebral artery
    D posterior cerebral artery
    E posterior inferior cerebellar artery

28. Of the following drugs the one which does not carry a risk of excacerbating asthma is

    A atenolol
    B diclofenac
    C co-proxamol
    D doxapram
    E tamoxifen

29. The following are signs of lateral medullary syndrome EXCEPT

    A diplopia
    B dissociated sensory loss
    C ipsilateral Horner's syndrome
    D nystagmus on looking to side of lesion
    E severe vertigo with vomiting

30. Risk factors for deep venous thrombosis include all of the following EXCEPT

   A alcoholic cirrhosis
   B antithrombin III deficiency
   C lupus anticoagulant
   D protein S deficiency
   E tobacco smoking

31. The following drugs may exacerbate psoriasis EXCEPT

   A alcohol
   B propranolol
   C quinine
   D terbinafine
   E thyroxine

32. Recognised features of Crohn's disease rather than ulcerative colitis include all of the following EXCEPT

   A rectal involvement when the colon is affected
   B pyoderma gangrenosum
   C nail clubbing
   D renal oxalate stones
   E uveitis

33. Recognised associations of ulcerative colitis rather than Crohn's disease include all of the following EXCEPT

   A amyloidosis
   B ankylosing spondylitis
   C hepatitis
   D ischiorectal abscess
   E sclerosing cholangitis

34. Bronchial malignancy is associated with exposure to all of the following substances EXCEPT

   A asbestos
   B chromium
   C coal dust
   D iron
   E iron oxides

35. Recognised features of anorexia nervosa include all of the following EXCEPT

   A constipation
   B hyperkalaemia
   C lanugo hair
   D primary amenorrhoea
   E sinus bradycardia

36. Erythema nodosum may be associated with infection with all of the following EXCEPT

   A *Borrelia burgdorferi*
   B chlamydia
   C leprosy
   D yersinia
   E tuberculosis

37. Finger clubbing may be associated with all of the following conditions EXCEPT

   A bronchiectasis
   B cirrhosis
   C coarctation of the aorta
   D coeliac disease
   E sarcoidosis

38. Irritable bowel syndrome is associated with all of the following EXCEPT

   A heart burn
   B greater prevalence in females
   C abdominal colic relieved by bowel opening
   D incomplete defecation
   E rectal mucus

39. Peripheral neuropathy may be associated with all of the following drugs EXCEPT

   A carbamazepine
   B isoniazid
   C metronidazole
   D nitrofurantoin
   E vincristine

40. Causes of atrial fibrillation include all of the following EXCEPT

   A cocaine intoxication
   B constrictive pericarditis
   C hyperthyroidism
   D mitral valve stenosis
   E myocardial ischaemia

41. Left atrial myxoma may present with all of the following EXCEPT

   A atrial fibrillation
   B increased ESR
   C mitral stenosis
   D pyrexia
   E weight loss

42. Osteoporosis is a recognised complication of each of the following EXCEPT

   A Addison's disease
   B long-term heparin usage
   C ovarian dysgenesis
   D primary biliary cirrhosis
   E thyrotoxicosis

43. Favourable points to note in critical reading appraisal of research papers are all of the following EXCEPT

   A a P value of <0.5
   B data with narrow confidence intervals
   C methods documenting selection criteria of subjects
   D use of case control studies for small numbers of subjects
   E use of randomised controlled trials

44. Epstein–Barr virus is linked with all of the following diseases EXCEPT

   A Burkitt's lymphoma
   B Hodgkin's lymphoma
   C infectious mononucleosis
   D nasopharyngeal carcinoma
   E sinonasal carcinoma

45. Turner's syndrome (gonadal dysgenesis) includes all of the following features EXCEPT

    A coarctation of the aorta
    B cubitus valgus
    C hyperconvex nails
    D lymphoedema of the feet
    E mental retardation

46. Central periumbilical abdominal pain features in all the following conditions EXCEPT

    A acute appendicitis
    B acute cholecystitis
    C acute pancreatitis
    D occlusion of the superior mesenteric artery
    E sickle-cell crisis

47. Clinical features of acromegaly may include all of the following EXCEPT

    A carpal tunnel syndrome
    B distal muscle weakness
    C goitre
    D hypertension
    E progressive heart failure

48. Painless haematuria is a characteristic feature of which ONE of the following conditions?

    A cystitis
    B hydronephrosis
    C renal papillary necrosis
    D renal artery stenosis
    E renal tuberculosis

49. Recognised causes of hypercalcaemia include all of the following EXCEPT

    A Conn's syndrome
    B thiazide diuretics
    C hyperparathyroidism
    D myeloma
    E sarcoidosis

50. The following statements are correct regarding amyloidosis
    EXCEPT

    A It is a soluble protein.
    B It is an extracellular protein.
    C It is arranged in beta-pleated configuration.
    D It is diagnosed by Congo red staining of a rectal biopsy.
    E It may be associated with multiple myeloma.

51. The following conditions are associated with conductive hearing loss
    EXCEPT

    A chronic secretory otitis media
    B Menière's disease
    C nasopharyngeal carcinoma
    D otosclerosis
    E perforation of the tympanic membrane

52. Paget's disease (osteitis deformans) is associated with all of the fol-
    lowing findings EXCEPT

    A hypocalcaemia
    B increased bone turnover
    C nerve deafness
    D pathological fractures
    E severe bone pain alleviated by intravenous disodium pamidronate

53. Non-articular manifestations of rheumatoid arthritis include all of
    the following EXCEPT

    A fibrosing alveolitis
    B keratoconjunctivitis sicca
    C nail bed infarcts
    D palmar erythema
    E peripheral neuropathy

54. Features commonly found in patients with portal hypertension
    include all of the following EXCEPT

    A ascites
    B encephalopathy
    C gastric varices
    D hypoglobulinaemia
    E splenomegaly

55. Steatorrhoea is a recognised feature of all of the following conditions EXCEPT

    A ankylostomiasis
    B coeliac disease
    C Crohn's disease
    D giardiasis
    E multiple jejunal diverticula

56. Recognised associations of coeliac disease (gluten-sensitive enteropathy) include all of the following EXCEPT

    A aphthous mouth ulcers
    B carcinoma of the oesophagus
    C dermatitis herpetiformis
    D HLA DR3
    E renal oxalate stones

57. Causes of wasting of the small muscles of the hand include all of the following EXCEPT

    A carpal tunnel syndrome
    B muscular dystrophy
    C myasthenia gravis
    D peripheral neuropathy
    E rheumatoid arthritis

58. Reflux oesophagitis may be caused by all of the following EXCEPT

    A anticholinergic drugs
    B *Helicobacter pylori*
    C hiatus hernia
    D post cardia surgery in achalasia
    E tricyclic antidepressants

59. Potential side-effects of phenothiazine-derived antipsychotic drugs include all of the following EXCEPT

    A diarrhoea
    B haemolytic anaemia
    C hypotension
    D neuroleptic malignant syndrome
    E tardive dyskinesia

60. Causes of monocular loss of vision include all of the following EXCEPT

    A carotid artery atheromatous plaque
    B disseminated sclerosis
    C epidural haematoma
    D subarachnoid haemorrhage
    E temporal arteritis

61. Metronidazole is used in the treatment of all of the following infectious EXCEPT

    A *Actinomycoces israelii*
    B bacterial vaginosis
    C giardiasis
    D *Helicobacter pylori*
    E leptospirosis

62. The following pairs of drug poisoning and antidotes are matched correctly EXCEPT

    A carbamazepine – activated charcoal
    B iron – dicobalt edetate
    C paracetamol – *N*-acetylcysteine
    D valium – flumazenil
    E warfarin – phytomenadione

63. Gout may be precipitated by all of the following EXCEPT

    A aspirin
    B excess exercise
    C purine-rich oily fish
    D surgery under local anaesthesia
    E thiazide diuretics

64. Non-metastatic effects of bronchial carcinoma include all of the following EXCEPT

    A hypercalcaemia
    B hypertrophic pulmonary osteoarthropathy
    C myasthenic syndrome
    D nephrotic syndrome
    E Terry's lines (white nails with pink tips)

65. Aortic regurgitation may be associated with each of the following EXCEPT

    A ankylosing spondylitis
    B aortic dissection
    C ASD ostium primum
    D infective endocarditis
    E Marfan's syndrome

66. Features of temporal lobe disease may include each of the following EXCEPT

    A aphasia
    B auditory hallucinations
    C automatism
    D olfactory hallucinations
    E upper homonymous quadrantanopsia

67. Acute cholecystitis may be associated with each of the following EXCEPT

    A absence of gallstones
    B absent bowel sounds
    C back pain
    D reflux oesophagitis
    E shoulder tip pain

68. The following statements regarding phaeochromocytoma are correct EXCEPT

    A It occurs in the adrenal medulla in the majority of cases.
    B It presents with glycosuria in the majority of cases.
    C It may require phenoxybenzamine and propranolol to control BP.
    D It may be autosomal dominantly inherited.
    E It is bilateral in 10% of cases.

69. Recognised features of SLE may include all of the following EXCEPT

    A anti-neutrophil cytoplasmic antibody positive
    B splenomegaly
    C normochromic normocytic anaemia
    D psychosis
    E rheumatoid factor positive

70. Haemolytic anaemia is a recognised complication of all of the following drugs EXCEPT

   A co-trimoxazole
   B dapsone
   C diclofenac
   D penicillin
   E pyridoxine

71. The following statements regarding coronary artery bypass graft (CABG) surgery are correct EXCEPT

   A CABG has greater efficacy than percutaneous transluminal coronary angioplasty (PTCA).
   B Graft patency rates with the left internal mammary artery are higher than with the saphenous vein.
   C Left main stem disease is a recognised indication.
   D Mortality rate is 5%.
   E Personality change is a recognised complication.

72. Tongue abnormalities are found in all of the following conditions EXCEPT

   A acromegaly
   B amyloidosis
   C CREST syndrome
   D motor neurone disease
   E vitamin B$_{12}$ deficiency

73. The following statements regarding hyperthyroidism are correct EXCEPT

   A Grave's disease accounts for the majority of cases.
   B Radioactive iodine has potential risks of hypoparathyroidism.
   C Severe cases may mimic acute abdomen.
   D There is an increased incidence among males.
   E Treatment is with carbimazole 20 mg bd for up to 1 year.

74. Recognised features of Marfan's syndrome include each of the following EXCEPT

   A aortic incompetence
   B autosomal dominant inheritance
   C lens dislocation
   D high arched palate
   E mental retardation

75. Recognised causes of portal hypertension include all of the following EXCEPT

    A inferior vena cava thrombosis
    B myelofibrosis
    C portal vein thrombosis
    D primary biliary cirrhosis
    E sarcoidosis

76. Potential complications of thiazide diuretics include each of the following EXCEPT

    A hypercalcaemia
    B hyperglycaemia
    C hyperuricaemia
    D intrahepatic cholestasis
    E metabolic acidosis

77. Recognised features of glandular fever (infectious mononucleosis) include all of the following EXCEPT

    A Bell's palsy
    B leukopenia
    C palatal petechiae
    D pericarditis
    E rash with administration of ampicillin

78. Gingival hypertrophy may be associated with all of the following EXCEPT

    A ciclosporin
    B lead poisoning
    C nifedipine
    D phenytoin
    E scurvy

79. Recognised features of Wernicke's encephalopathy include all of the following EXCEPT

    A altered consciousness
    B ataxic gait
    C external rectus ophthalmoplegia
    D horizontal nystagmus
    E ptosis

80. The following tumour markers and tumours are correctly matched EXCEPT

   A alkaline phosphatase – prostate carcinoma
   B alpha-fetoprotein – choriocarcinoma
   C CA-125 – ovarian carcinoma
   D CA-19.9 – pancreatic carcinoma
   E human chorionic gonadotrophin – hydatidiform mole

81. Recognised complications of diabetes mellitus include each of the following EXCEPT

   A loss of libido
   B orthostatic hypotension
   C nephrotic syndrome
   D nocturnal diarrhoea
   E vomiting

82. Features of temporal arteritis (giant cell arteritis) may include all of the following EXCEPT

   A bitemporal hemianopsia
   B dysarthria
   C elevated ESR
   D jaw claudication
   E scalp tenderness

83. Recognised causes of amyloidosis include each of the following EXCEPT

   A bronchiectasis
   B cirrhosis
   C multiple myeloma
   D osteomyelitis
   E rheumatoid arthritis

84. Features of polymyalgia rheumatica (PMR) may include all of the following EXCEPT

   A angina
   B depression
   C hypopituitarism
   D morning stiffness involving the proximal muscles
   E pulmonary infarct

85. The following hypersensitivity reactions and examples are correctly matched EXCEPT

A Type I – idiopathic thrombocytopenic purpura
B Type I – urticaria
C Type II – ABO incompatibility
D Type II – Goodpasture's syndrome
E Type IV– tuberculosis

86. Features of pure mitral stenosis include all of the following EXCEPT

A haemoptysis
B left parasternal heave
C left ventricular hypertrophy
D loud first heart sound
E mid-diastolic murmur at the apex

87. The following statements regarding typhoid fever are correct EXCEPT

A It has a mortality rate of 10% if left untreated.
B It is caused by *Salmonella typhi*.
C It may be complicated by osteomyelitis.
D It presents with abdominal pain and bloody diarrhoea.
E Rose spots occur in 40% of patients.

88. Scant body hair is ONLY associated with

A anorexia nervosa
B Cushing's syndrome
C Klinefelter's syndrome
D panhypopituitarism
E Turner's syndrome

89. Pernicious anaemia is associated with all of the following EXCEPT

A increased incidence of pancreatic carcinoma
B jaundice
C mental confusion
D myxoedema
E splenomegaly

90. Hepatitis A infection is associated with all of the following EXCEPT

   A an incubation period of up to 6 weeks
   B eating shellfish
   C faecal–oral route of transmission
   D jaundice in the majority of cases
   E presence of IgM antibody in recent infection

91. Tropical disease infection is associated with coma in all of the following conditions EXCEPT

   A malaria
   B rabies
   C schistosomiasis
   D trypanosomiasis
   E typhoid fever

92. Primary biliary cirrhosis may be associated with all of the following EXCEPT

   A dry eyes
   B night blindness
   C presence of antimitochondrial antibody
   D raised liver copper in the early stages
   E raised serum IgM levels

93. Neuropathic (Charcot's) joints may be found in all of the following conditions EXCEPT

   A cauda equina lesion
   B leprosy
   C tabes dorsalis
   D syringomyelia
   E multiple sclerosis

94. A pedestrian involved in a RTA fails to regain consciousness. Possible causes include all of the following EXCEPT

   A cardiac tamponade
   B extradural haematoma
   C fat embolism
   D myocardial infarction
   E pneumothorax

95. Vitamin B$_{12}$ deficiency may result from all of the following conditions EXCEPT

    A Crohn's disease
    B coeliac disease
    C diphyllobothriasis
    D giardiasis
    E jejunal diverticulosis

96. Immune complex mediated diseases include all of the following EXCEPT

    A diabetes mellitus
    B Goodpasture's syndrome
    C primary biliary cirrhosis
    D Rhesus incompatibility
    E SLE

97. X-linked diseases include all of the following conditions EXCEPT

    A achondroplasia
    B Christmas disease
    C Duchenne's muscular dystrophy
    D hypophosphataemic rickets
    E retinitis pigmentosa

98. The following statements are correct regarding *Helicobacter pylori* EXCEPT

    A It has a predilection for the gastric antrum.
    B It is a Gram-negative organism.
    C It is isolated in more patients with gastric rather than duodenal ulcers.
    D It may be asymptomatic at the time of infection.
    E It produces urease.

99. The following statistical definitions are true EXCEPT

    A A negatively skewed distribution is one in which the mean is greater than the median.
    B Standard deviation indicates what interval, measured from the mean, includes 34% of all observations in a normal distribution.
    C The median is the middle score of an ordered frequency distribution.
    D The mode is the value which occurs most frequently in the distribution.
    E The variance is the average of the sum of the square deviations.

100. The following statements regarding hepatitis C virus are correct EXCEPT

A Infection is preventable with passive immunisation.
B It is characterised by a mild acute infection.
C It more often progresses to a chronic hepatitis than hepatitis B.
D It may be transmitted through shared toothbrushes.
E It may be transmitted via blood transfusions.

Answers to Paper Ten BOFs

Criterion Referencing Marks

* – 25–50% of candidates expected to get correct
** – 50–75% of candidates expected to get correct
*** – 75–100% of candidates expected to get correct

The notional PASS MARK is 71%

1. A **

2. E ***

3. D *** Erythropoietin is produced in the kidney.

4. D ***

5. C ** Hepatitis B is a DNA virus. The incubation period is up to 6 months. HbeAg indicates high infectivity. Carrier status exists if the HbsAg is present for >6 months.

6. D ***

7. C *

8. E ** Thrombophlebitis migrans may be associated with cancer of the pancreas. Other cutaneous manifestations of malignancy include acanthosis nigricans and dematomyositis.

9. D ** HbA1C is usually monitored every 3–6 months.

10. C ***

11. C *

12. E * Phytophotodermatitis is caused by chromophobe furocoumarins (plants) and results in a linear skin eruption 1–2 days post-exposure to the plant and UVA. Poison ivy results in contact dermatitis.

13. A * Melanoma has a worse prognosis if it is in the BANS area (back, arms, neck or scalp).

14. A ***

15. A ** Cyclophosphamide and not ciclosporin may cause diffuse pulmonary fibrosis.

16. D *** A left parasternal heave is associated with pulmonary stenosis. Aortic stenosis is characterised by a basal systolic murmur.

17. C *** Serum calcium and phosphate levels are normal, but alkaline phosphatase is characteristically raised.

18. D ***

19. C ** Acute renal failure is also associated with hyponatraemia and hyperkalaemia.

20. E **

21. E ***

22. A ***

23. C *** Retinal detachment is more common in myopics.

24. D **

25. C *** Peripheral neuropathy may be associated with hypothyroidism.

26. A ***

27. E ***

28. D ** NSAIDs and beta-blockers are contraindicated in asthma. The dextropropoxyphene content of co-proxamol will cause respiratory depression in overdose only. Tamoxifen can cause an idiosyncratic reaction.

29. A **

30. E **

31. E ** Psoriasis may be exacerbated by antimalarials, beta-blockers, lithium, NSAIDs and stress.

32. A ***

33. D ***

34. C **

35. B *** Anorexia nervosa may result in hypokalaemia.

36. A ** Erythema nodosum may also occur with infections with streptococcus.

37. E **

38. A ***

39. A ** Phenytoin may also cause peripheral neuropathy.

40. A ***

41. C **

42. A ***

43. A ** A *P* value of <0.05 is desirable and indicates significance in clinical research.

44. E **

45. E **

46. B ***

47. B ** Acromegaly is associated with proximal muscle wasting.

48. E **

49. A **

50. A *

51. B **

52. A *** Paget's disease is associated with normal calcium and phosphate levels.

53. E *

54. D ***

55. A **

56. E ** Other associations of coeliac disease include anaemia, osteomalacia, GI lymphoma, growth retardation and gastric carcinoma.

57. C ***

58. B **

59. A *

60. D *

61. E **

62. B *** The antidote for iron poisoning is desferrioxamine.

63. D ** Gout may also be precipitated by obesity and secondarily by leukaemia, polycythaemia and renal failure.

64. E ** Leuconychia is associated with cirrhosis.

65. C ***

66. E ** Olfactory hallucinations may result from damage to the medial temporal lobe or the uncus.

67. D *** Jaundice may result from the coexistence of common bile duct stones.

68. B ** 30% of cases present with glycosuria.

69. A ** Positive ANCA is associated with Wegener's granulomatosis. Positive ANA is associated with SLE.

70. E ** Pyridoxine is a form of treatment for haemolytic anaemia. Co-trimoxazole contains sulfamethoxazole. Another drug associated with haemolytic anaemia is sulfadiazine.

71. D ** The mortality for CABG operations is less than 2%.

72. C **

73. D **

74. E ***

75. A **

76. E ***

77. B *** Infectious mononucleosis is associated with lymphocytosis and a positive monospot test. Ampicillin and amoxicillin should be avoided.

78. B **

79. D * Wernicke's encephalopathy results from thiamine deficiency and is associated with vertical nystagmus, ophthalmoplegia and ataxia.

80. A ***

81. A ***

82. A *** Temporal arteritis is associated with monocular blindness.

83. B **

84. A **

85. A * ITP is an example of a Type II (cytotoxic) hypersensitivity reaction.

86. C ***

87. D ***

88. D **

89. A *** Pernicious anaemia is a risk factor for gastric carcinoma.

90. D ***

91. C **

92. D ***

93. E **

94. E ***

95. B **

96. D **

97. A **

98. C *** Most patients with a duodenal ulcer harbour this organism.

99. A **

100. A *** Hepatitis C virus is associated with an increased risk of hepatocellular carcinoma and more than 50% develop chronic hepatitis.

dexapram
amyotrophic lateral sclerosis